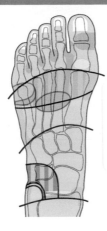

Reflex

D0707781

of the Feet

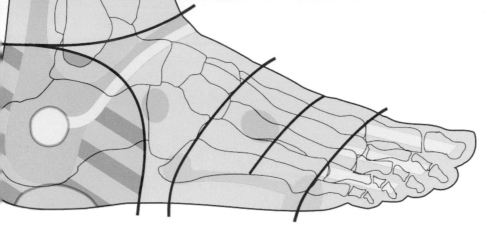

Reflex Zone Therapy of the Feet

A COMPREHENSIVE GUIDE FOR HEALTH PROFESSIONALS

HANNE MARQUARDT

Translated by
Ann Callard Lett

Revised edition translated
by Nikolas Win Myint

Healing Arts Press
Rochester, Vermont • Toronto, Canada

Healing Arts Press
One Park Street
Rochester, Vermont 05767
www.HealingArtsPress.com

Healing Arts Press is a division of Inner Traditions International

Originally published in German under the title *Reflexzonenarbeit am FUB* by Karl F. Haug
    Verlag in MVS Medizinverlage Stuttgart GmbH & Co KG Germany
First German edition published in 1975. 23rd edition published in 2007
First English edition published in 1983 by Thorsons Publishers Limited
First U.S. edition published in 1984 by Healing Arts Press
Revised U.S. edition published in 2011 by Healing Arts Press

Note to the reader: *This book is intended as an informational guide. The remedies,
approaches, and techniques described herein are meant to supplement, and not to be a substitute for, professional medical care or treatment. They should not be used to treat a serious
ailment without prior consultation with a qualified health care professional.*

Library of Congress Cataloging-in-Publication Data

Marquardt, Hanne.
   [Reflexzonenarbeit am Fuss. English]
   Reflex zone therapy of the feet : a comprehensive guide for health professionals / Hanne
Marquardt ; translated from the German by Ann Callard Lett; revised edition translated
from the German by Nikolas Win Myint. — Rev. U.S. ed.
      p. ; cm.
   Includes bibliographical references and index.
   Summary: "The classic reflexology reference with new material and new illustrations"—
Provided by publisher.
   ISBN 978-1-59477-361-7
   1. Reflexotherapy. 2. Foot—Massage. I. Title.
   [DNLM: 1. Reflexotherapy—methods. 2. Foot. WB 962]
   RM723.R43M3713 2011
   615.8'224—dc22

                                                           2010028271

Printed and bound in India by Replika Press Pvt. Ltd.

10 9 8 7 6 5 4 3 2 1

Text design and layout by Virginia Scott Bowman
This book was typeset in Garamond Premier Pro with Life, Copperplate, and Gill Sans as
display typefaces

Contents

Preface to
the New Edition

For almost fifty years, the feet have been the professional center of my life, and I note with satisfaction that reflexology of the feet has become well accepted as a physical form of therapy during that time. Today, it is among the best-known methods of complementary medicine and has contributed its part to bringing medical science and traditional healing methods into greater harmony.

Increasingly, people realize that the feet play a "load-bearing" role not only in therapeutic settings, but in day-to-day life. When people feel the ground "shifting under their feet," this type of therapy is all the more relevant. Moreover, this solid approach of working by hand is now frequently seen as a necessary counterbalance to our technology-driven lifestyles. People feel that touch is an essential need that has effects on both physical and emotional levels. A disabled child I was treating, who I thought would not understand the nature of this therapy, told me: "I understand what you are doing—you are treating my roots."

There were several reasons for my detailed reworking and expanding of this new edition:

1. The time had come to more closely look at a number of apparent contradictions related to the location of the reflexology zones. The more simple mapping of the reflex zones that I learned in 1958 from

the transmittal of the knowledge of William Fitzgerald and Eunice Ingham were for me the basis for our training methods. But this is a living form of therapy that continues to develop and adapt to the needs of its times. As such, while the more simple basis from which it developed is not "wrong," I think it is helpful to add further explanation.

2. Although it went largely unnoticed, I continued to change and expand the location of the original zones in previous editions as well. While the zones are illustrated and discussed in more detail in the 1993 version of my book *Praktischen Lehrbuch der Reflexzonentherapie am Fuss* [*Practical Handbook of Foot Reflexology*], published by Hippokrates Publishers, in this book I want to keep to the style of the more simple illustrations. The main changes in location relate to four zones: the pituitary gland, the bladder, the knee, and the solar plexus—all of which I mark and explain in the text and illustrations.

3. I have replaced the previous term *causal reflexology zones* with the more appropriate term *background zones*. This term is less binding and has been used in all my work since the publication of the official teaching guide (including translations into other languages). Like its predecessor, this term refers to the possible causal background of symptoms with which patients present themselves for treatment.

4. The notion of "similar shapes," which has been very important to the continued development of foot reflexology since the early 1990s, continues to be easily recognizable in the simpler illustrations. This idea suggests that because a flexed foot is similar in shape to the body of a seated person, the foot can then be treated as an actual mirror of each person's body. The relation between the sitting person and the surprisingly precise "smaller mirror" in his feet is clearly visible, and furnishes a reliable therapeutic guide.

5. Since different developments in the health system have given rise to

the recognition that we are all also responsible for our own health, I want to note in this edition that while in principle every person can treat their own feet as well as those of others, there is an important **distinction between therapy and health maintenance** in the sense of prevention. (See indications for specialists and nonspecialists, p. 29–30) In brief,

The treatment of ill people should be carried out by trained medical-therapeutic specialists, as called for by law.

Nonspecialists can treat feet to **maintain health and wellness,** and to treat **healthy people** suffering from minor everyday ailments.

The revised version of this book will continue to be a helpful entry into this field for interested medical specialists, allowing them to treat individual zones and see the therapeutic effects on their patients.

At the same time, the book is also intended for private individuals who—while keeping to the limits identified above—will find in this a reliable guide to treating themselves, their families, and their friends. Given the increased recognition of people's responsibility for their own health, recent years have seen an increased interest by health-conscious people in this type of therapy, which uses one's own healing powers to treat root causes, rather than focusing on suppressing symptoms.

I hope that the changes and improvements in this new edition will contribute to bringing clarity to the application of this valuable and comprehensive therapy. Those who recognize and practice within its limits will find it a broad framework with many possibilities.

HANNE MARQUARDT
KÖNIGSFELD-BURGBERG, GERMANY

Note: In the interest of readability, the present work does not always refer explicitly to both male and female genders, though whenever one is cited, this is intended as also including the other.

Translator's Preface

TO THE FIRST ENGLISH EDITION, 1983

This is the first authoritative manual on reflex zone therapy of the feet to come into English print since Eunice Ingham's books—*Stories the Feet Can Tell* and *Stories the Feet Have Told*—were published in the late 1930s. A very great deal has been added to our knowledge of the subject since that time through the work done by Hanne Marquardt and her colleagues.

Several of the treatments mentioned in this book are better known on the Continent than they are in some English-speaking countries. However, a growing interest in alternative medicine is already well under way, including a reassessment of what is practical and useful in allopathic medicine and curiosity about the roles that can be played by some traditional and less well-known methods. Those who care for the sick are under a continuing obligation to look anew at ways of alleviating the pain and disability of their patients.

After twenty-five years as a nurse, midwife, ward sister, and tutor in England and South Africa, I became acquainted with reflex zone therapy after a serious personal accident, and subsequently attended the introductory and advanced courses at Hanne Marquardt's school in Germany. Courses are now being held in the United Kingdom, and it is hoped that with the publication of this book more people will come to know something of this interesting and valuable work.

Reflex zone therapy is not a panacea for all ills; practitioners require disciplined application to become skilled at obtaining the best results. The uses to which this therapy can be put are many; practiced well, it will assist many people.

This book is a translation. I have tried to convey the ideas and explanations given by Hanne Marquardt in a form that will be understood and received by a lay and professional English-speaking public. Any errors of interpretation must be mine alone, yet I trust that the book is true to the spirit and practice of reflex zone therapy as taught by Hanne Marquardt.

ANN CALLARD LETT,
PRINCIPAL, BRITISH SCHOOL OF
REFLEX ZONE THERAPY OF THE FEET,
LONDON

Foreword

TO THE FIRST EDITION, 1975
BY DR. ERICH RAUCH

I was introduced to reflex zone therapy of the feet through reading Eunice Ingham's original book *Stories the Feet Can Tell* in 1965. My interest was sufficiently roused to pursue the subject further, and my colleagues and I began to examine the feet of most of our patients and, where it seemed appropriate, to treat them. After hundreds of such cases, there remained no doubt in our minds that the accounts given by Mrs. Ingham, and the discoveries made by Dr. William Fitzgerald, author of *Zone Therapy*, were factual, impartial, verifiable, and medically sound—not illusory.

Numerous areas of the feet lie in a particular reflex relationship and connection to identifiable zones of the body and its organs. This is a help in both diagnosis and treatment, as can readily be proven. The feet— seldom submitted to therapy, usually fitted into tight shoes, and rarely exposed to the air—may now, thanks to Dr. Fitzgerald and Mrs. Ingham, become the effective starting point for the treatment of innumerable conditions.

Understandably, many of our patients were initially skeptical and even bewildered when we began to massage their feet. Those who saw no connection between their ailments and treatment of their feet were particularly perplexed.

Today, due to the renaissance of interest in acupuncture, there is a growing readiness to believe that interrelationships exist between certain points of the body and organs widely removed from such points. Due to the wide lay acceptance of acupuncture, a similar relationship between certain areas of the feet and organs lying at some distance from these areas is now at least open to question. The concomitant feelings of sensitivity and well-being—which pervade the whole body in accompaniment to a massage of the reflex zones of the feet, and the therapy's undoubted efficacy, have been instrumental in bringing about this change in a short space of time.

At this stage we first learned that courses of instruction in reflex zone therapy of the feet were being held. Mrs. Hanne Marquardt, the author of this book, who had learned the method from Eunice Ingham and made it her specialty, invited us to one of these. This introductory course was most instructive. It proved again how little manual dexterity could be learned from a book alone, and brought into view the breadth and scope of the practice, and its wide range of application. Results showed themselves soon afterward in a remarkable improvement in therapeutic effect. It was thus small wonder that reflex zone therapy of the feet established for itself a wholly scientific place among those of us studying holistic medicine.

In particular, Mrs. Marquardt proved the value of treatment of the feet for such a wide range of ailments that it has since become a quite indispensable form of treatment among us for disorders of the musculoskeletal system and the spine; functional disorders of the respiratory and genitourinary systems; developmental disorders of childhood; and several others. Many rare conditions are amenable to treatment with this method provided that their reflex signature has been visibly and palpably engraved on the relevant foot zone.

Our combined experience in this field has left us in no doubt that a method as effective as this requires that those who wish to practice should have the necessary basic knowledge, and sufficient practical and theoretical training. Mrs. Marquardt, in every sense the fit and proper person to train pupils in this discipline, strongly recommends several training courses. Aspiring practitioners should nevertheless have had some previous training and experience in working with the sick, either in nursing, physiotherapy, or some related discipline, and they should have undergone a series of reflex zone massages of the feet.

Despite the merits of this form of treatment, it is possible to introduce errors into its practice. A therapist working without due care will bring the patient a less effective form of treatment, and disrepute upon the method. One can only be warned against those who set up training courses without relevant experience. Those who would truly learn must shun bad teachers. The many mechanical aids that have appeared in recent times and have been widely promoted must also be avoided. There is no fundamental justification for the claims made on their behalf, nor do they satisfy any medical criteria. They do not permit the right application of pressure or the right touch.

A prerequisite for this work is a good working relationship with a doctor, at best with one who has an understanding of the subject. Therein lie the interests of the patient, the therapist, and not least of all, the method.

Finally, it must be said that among all the medical sciences there is not one form of therapy that does not have its boundaries. Reflex zone therapy of the feet is no exception. It should not be practiced indiscriminately, nor with all one's critical faculties suspended. Its practice must be governed by awareness of its scope and limitations. It is irresponsible and unethical to raise false hopes.

We find the evaluation of abnormal findings in the feet particularly important. It matters not whether they are recognized through means of sight, touch, or painful reactions they may provoke in the patient. There are four possible causes to be considered when these abnormal findings are encountered:

1. Temporary functional overload of the organ related to that zone—for example, in the heart zone immediately after a severe heart attack, in the liver after a fatty meal, in the zones relating to the eyes after a long car journey, and so forth.
2. Slight or insignificant dysfunction of an organ. Current clinical tests cannot as yet assess with accuracy such damage. This is

referred to as damage to the tissues that has not yet become consciously or clinically manifest. The diagnostic techniques of Dr. F. X. Mayr—such as electroacupuncture, impulse dermography, and so on—need to be brought into wider use in conjunction with this therapy to provide a more accurate diagnosis of such dysfunction.

3. Functional disease of the organ related to that zone.
4. Systemic disease involving that organ.

Abnormal reflex zones should not therefore be interpreted as indicating disease, nor provide the basis for making an "interesting" diagnosis. Diagnosis is the prerogative of the doctor. When a doctor is familiar with this method, he will certainly take into account diagnostic indications arising from abnormal zones on the feet and will find them a worthy adjunct in drawing up a differential diagnosis.

There is often a great temptation to lay too much emphasis on the abnormal reflex zones found, particularly when the patient asks what this or that painful area signifies. A good practitioner, whose sole interest is the patient's progress, will only allude to the possibility of malfunction of organs or systems in that zone, and not declare the presence of specific disease. The therapist will not therefore create anxiety or a neurotic response in a patient who has a hypochondriacal tendency.

Above all else, *Nil Nocere!*—Do No Harm—remains the maxim of all healing disciplines. I direct all those who wish to practice reflex zone therapy of the feet to reflect on this statement and to base their work upon it.

The publication of this book has met a great need. The author, Hanne Marquardt, has given within its covers expression to all the results of her training in this specialty arising from her knowledge and practical experience. She has laid the necessary foundation for all who are interested in the practice of reflex zone therapy of the feet. The practical knowledge she has acquired and her dedicated concern over the years have led reflex zone therapy of the feet to its properly recognized place alongside other manual therapies. The many do-it-yourself methods that have developed recently are something of a threat to this recognition. When the therapist truly endeavors to understand all that is embraced in this method, both therapist and patient will find joy in its practice, and unanticipated success will often be the result.

I hope that this book finds a wide audience, and wish for the author and her numerous readers and pupils, much success.

DR. ERICH RAUCH
MARIA WORTH/KARNETERN, W. GERMANY

Erich Rauch, M.D., a physician specializing in natural therapies, has been the director of a large and successful health spa in Austria for many years. He is the author of numerous books on detoxification, hydrotherapy, resistance-strengthening measures, and naturopathy.

Introduction

TO THE FIRST EDITION, 1975

In the summer of 1958, while working as a massage therapist in a sanatorium in southern Germany, I discovered a book called *Stories the Feet Can Tell,* written by Eunice Ingham in 1938. More from a sense of curiosity toward an unknown subject than out of a spirit of scientific investigation, I began to try out this unusual method of treatment. I took every available foot into my hands, palpated, observed, massaged, and compared them, until I was myself persuaded that the feet represented a central switchboard, from where—I knew not how or why—observable effects over the whole of the body could be provoked.

What had begun as a nonserious curiosity in my spare time then gave place to a serious preoccupation. The therapeutic results of my massages to the feet, amateurish as they then were, encouraged me and surprised my patients. After nine years of being engrossed with the reflex zones of the feet, I finally came to meet and work with Eunice Ingham, then already eighty years old, but full of vitality, and moreover, a percipient massage therapist in the United States. (Sadly, she died in December 1974.)

My earlier training as a nurse in England served me well, as it gave me the background knowledge and understanding of the language, which I needed. This thoroughly useful and worthwhile beginning stimulated me to think continually about the development of the method, and at the same time I began to approach other interested and professional specialists. An experimental first training course in reflex zone therapy of the feet was embarked upon despite the difficulties:

1

- Transposing a method from the United States, land of "limitless opportunities," to Europe, with its more cautious outlook
- Adapting to modern needs a method of treatment whose meaning had been grasped at the beginning of the twentieth century, and which claimed to alleviate a diversity of illnesses
- Explaining this form of treatment, which was as yet not understood scientifically, though it had been developed and refined to such a degree that it could now be taught to experienced manual therapists

The venture prospered. After this first attempt, numerous courses of instruction took place over the subsequent years. There have been invitations from medical professional circles to lecture and instruct in Austria, Switzerland, England, South Africa, and Israel.

Meanwhile, qualified students who have attended courses in reflex zone therapy of the feet are working in twenty-six countries in Europe and abroad. In 1972 a branch school was started in Denmark for the Scandinavian countries. The ground was prepared for an English-speaking subsidiary school in Johannesburg, South Africa, in 1975, and affiliated schools now exist in Britain and Israel. Several large hospitals are discovering the potential of this method and proving through experience the value of reflex zone therapy of the feet. Walter Froneberg, who is particularly interested in manual therapies relating to the nervous system, showed that there are reflex zones in the feet relating to the central and autonomic nervous systems; he is working closely with the school here in Germany to further elucidate and expand our knowledge.

This book is the result of fruitful work done by my students and patients. Over the years it has become evident that an account of all the knowledge handed down and all newly acquired information should be amalgamated in book form.

In the years to come, I wish for reflex zone therapy of the feet the same vitality in its total growth as has been evident until now. With faith and gratitude I wish to pass on to "faithful hands" all that I know and have learned as a result of my experiences; may they further this knowledge and work.

PART ONE

THEORY

1

The History of
Reflex Zone Therapy

Dr. William Fitzgerald, the founder of Zone Therapy, was born in Middletown, Connecticut, in 1872. He graduated with a degree in medicine from the University of Vermont in 1895, and then spent some years in hospitals in Vienna, Paris, and London. He later practiced in the Hospital for Diseases of the Ear, Nose and Throat in Hartford, Connecticut, then transferred his practice and teaching to New York. He died in Stamford, Connecticut, in 1942.

Developing the work of Dr. Harry Bressler, Dr. Fitzgerald came to Vienna in the early years of this century to consider the possibility of treating organs through pressure points. In his book *Zone Therapy,* he makes some interesting remarks about its history:

> A form of treatment by means of pressure points was known in India and China 5,000 years ago. This knowledge appears however to have been lost or forgotten. Perhaps it was set aside in favour of acupuncture, which emerged as the stronger growth from the same root.[1]

In central European countries similar methods were described in 1582 by Dr. Adamus and Dr. A'Tatis. At about the same time Dr. Ball of Leipzig published a manuscript on the treatment of separate organs of the body by means of pressure points. The great Florentine sculptor, Cellini

(1500–1571), used strong pressure on his fingers and toes to relieve pain anywhere in his body, with remarkable success.

The twentieth American president, James A. Garfield (1831–1881), was able to alleviate the pains he had following an assassination attempt by applying pressure to various points in his feet. No other pain-killing medicines gave him relief.

The relationship between reflex points and the internal organs of the body was known by various North American Indian tribes and used in the treatment of disease. This knowledge has been preserved over many centuries and is still used on Indian reservations for the relief of pain.

Evidently, sick people—at least in Europe, Asia, and America—have intuitively discovered numerous points where pressure could be applied to bring about certain known effects on other parts of the body, and have used them in the relief of their diseases. Those who today invoke the involuntary gestures of biting their teeth together, clenching their fists, or spontaneously applying pressure to an acutely painful area may well be employing relics of a similar background.

In 1916, Dr. Edwin F. Bowers first publicly described the treatment propounded by Dr. Fitzgerald and called it "Zone Therapy." One year later their combined work appeared in the book *Zone Therapy*.[2] It contained therapeutic proposals and recommendations for doctors, dentists, gynecologists, E.N.T. specialists, and chiropractors. According to Dr. George Starr White in 1925, "the fact that today Zone Therapy is probably known more widely throughout the United States and all places where magazines and newspapers are printed than any other single method of therapy, proves that the foundation of this work is solid."

Dr. Fitzgerald gave courses of instruction and gathered about him a circle of practitioners. Diagrams of the zones of the feet and the corresponding division of the ten zones of the body appeared in the first edition of his book. It is likely that in creating these, he was drawing on aspects of Native American folk medicine that were familiar to him. His contribution was to identify and thus open to therapeutic use relationships and countereffects between parts of the body and its whole.

The groundwork had thus been laid when the American massage

therapist, Eunice Ingham, started her training in this discipline. She spent years gaining insight into the manner of its working. The diagrams and accounts of those around her, allied to her own practical observation, served to form the basis for her "pressure massage" of the feet. As a result of this wide experience, Eunice Ingham played her part in putting the practice she called *"Reflexology"* on its "feet," concentrating her attention and knowledge on the small surfaces of the foot.

She developed a special, subtle method of massage, which she called the Ingham Method of compression massage, described in her book *Stories the Feet Can Tell.*[3] Her original massage, performed "as though one was refining sugar crystals in one's hand," was continually being altered and improved during her many years of practice and is now taught as the cornerstone of this work at our present state of knowledge.

Between 1958 and 1967, I successfully used reflex zone therapy in my own practice, and since 1967 each new development has been tested at the School for Reflex Zone Therapy by fully qualified trained workers from all medical and therapeutic professions.

Thus, the method has behind it, as do many others, a gradual development. Through many centuries, it has passed from being an old, intuitive folk medicine to its present adaptable form of manual therapy, by means of which the present generation can be helped.

2

The Zone Grid

The practice of reflex zone therapy of the feet is derived from two basic concepts: (1) the division of the body into ten vertical zones, postulated by Dr. William Fitzgerald, and (2) the corresponding ten-zone grid of the feet, in which are dovetailed the reflex zones, which have been known empirically for centuries.

THE ZONES OF THE BODY

The foundation of reflex zone therapy divides the body into both vertical and horizontal zones.

The Ten Vertical Body Zones

The body is divided into ten equal, vertical zones by imaginary lines drawn through the head, arms, trunk, and feet. These zones incorporate all the organs of the head and trunk. It is not clear what basis Dr. Fitzgerald used for this division, though there are hypotheses that these vertical fields depict stylized and simplified meridians. This interpretation, and the coordination of these fields, is mentioned in the early American writings.

This vertical division of the body is useful to us for work on the reflex zones of the feet, as it provides an anatomical-topographical aid, such as that used to divide the globe by meridians.

The Three Transverse Body Zones

Whereas the ten vertical zones only allow us to locate the organs of the body in their longitudinal relationship to one another, we realized in 1970, as a result of our studies in the school, that these vertical lines could be transected by similarly imagined horizontal lines, which divide the body into transverse zones. These imaginary lines were then related to the skeleton. We found that, in practice, three lines sufficed for this division, and they could be related to well-known anatomical landmarks. The first line is in the upper region of the shoulder girdle; the second line is in the region of the lower costal margin—the waistline; and the third is at the level of the pelvic floor.

These three transverse zones are shown in figure 1.

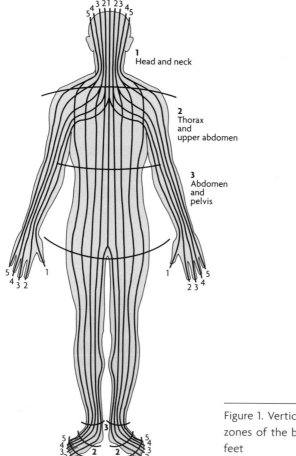

Figure 1. Vertical and transverse zones of the body and the feet

With the help of this vertical-horizontal framework, the organs of the body are found lying in one of its three main compartments:

- The structures of the head and neck lie above the horizontal line drawn along the shoulder girdle.
- The thorax and upper abdomen with their organs lie within the region bounded by the horizontal lines of the shoulder girdle above and the waistline below.
- The organs of the abdomen and pelvis lie within the region bounded by the horizontal lines of the waistline above and the pelvic floor below.

THE ZONE GRID ON THE FEET

For the purposes of reflex zone massage to the feet, there are distinct relationships between the body zones and the reflex zones on the feet.

The Vertical Zones

The vertical zones divide the feet from heel to toe into ten fields, which correspond to the ten zones of the body and their organs. Generally, the reflex zone of an organ occupies the same vertical zone in the feet as it does in the body, and should be looked for there.

For example, the right shoulder girdle—vertical zones 4 and 5 on the right side of the body—finds its corresponding foot reflex zone in the same fourth and fifth vertical zones around the joint of the small toe on the right foot. (See figures 2a and 2b on pages 10–11.)

The left kidney—in vertical body zones 2 and 3 on the left—has its reflex zone in the vertical zones 2 and 3 of the left foot, in the region of the proximal end of the second and third metatarsal bones.

Similarly, the spine, which is located in vertical body zone 1 on the right and left sides of the body, is reflected in zone 1 of the feet—that is to say along the longitudinal arch of both soles.

In the same way, all the organs of the body find their reflex zones on the feet in the corresponding vertical zone.

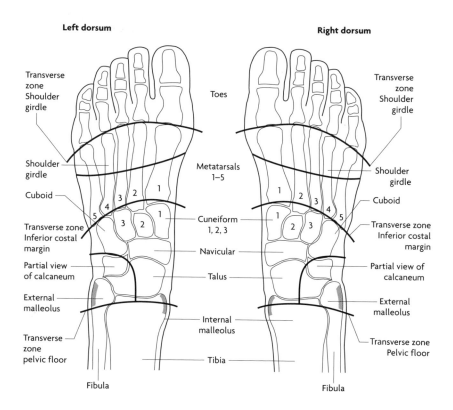

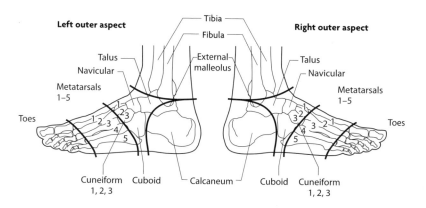

Figure 2a. The bones of the foot and the three transverse zones

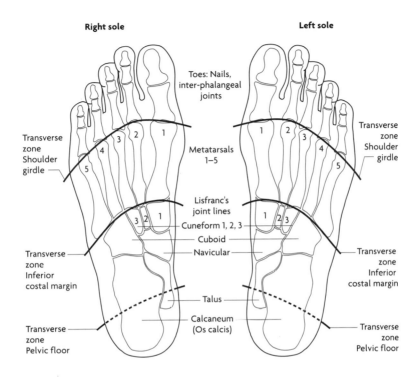

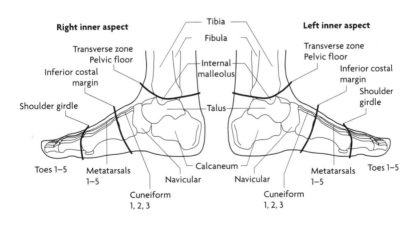

Figure 2b. The bones of the foot and the three transverse zones

The Three Transverse Zones

The three transverse zones are employed in the same fashion to divide the feet; they represent not only the division of the feet, but also a division of the body into three parts. These are easily recognized because of their correlation to anatomical features, as follows.

The first transverse line of the foot passes through the metatarso-phalangeal joints, and corresponds to the transverse line at the level of the shoulder girdle. Therefore, the reflex zones of the structures of the head and neck are found in the phalanges of the toes.

Reflex zones for the organs and structures of the thorax and upper abdomen are found in the anatomical region of the metatarsal bones on both feet and are bounded by Lisfranc's joint line (along which partial amputation of the foot is customarily performed). This second transverse line corresponds to the transverse division of the body at the waistline.

Reflex zones for the organs and structures of the abdomen and pelvis are found in the area of the tarsal bones, up to and including the inner and outer malleoli. This third transverse line corresponds to the line on the body at the level of the pelvic floor and hip joint.

By dividing the feet into imaginary vertical and transverse zones, we construct a grid into which each zone fits like a chip of stone into a mosaic. Based on our experience, the vertical zones usually divide the body equally and bilaterally as they run from head to foot and do not cross over in the neck. In some cases, the zones may shift slightly to the left or to the right; instructions for dealing with such cases are discussed in my book *Praktischen Lehrbuch des Reflexzonentherapie am Fuss* [*Practical instructions for foot reflexology*].[1]

The Concept
of Reflex Zones

The term *reflex zone* has long been used in manual therapies, most frequently in connection with neurological reflexes. Connective tissue massage has also been described as "work in the reflectory zones of the connective tissue."[1] At the end of the nineteenth century, Henry Head and James Mackenzie had already described such reflectory relationships between the periphery of the body and its internal organs.

According to the medical dictionary of Dr. W. Pschyrembel, the word *reflex* in the strict medical sense means "an involuntary muscle contraction due to an external stimulus and relayed by a central organ such as the spinal cord."[2] In the context of reflex zones of the feet, the word *reflex* is not used in this sense, but has two other meanings:

1. As reflecting the entire organism (head, neck, and trunk) on a small screen (the feet), rather like a reflex camera
2. Referring to characteristic sections of the feet, which have been shown empirically to have a direct energy relationship with the internal organs

These definitions of *reflex* have nothing to do with Head and Mackenzie, or with connective tissue massage, or the energy network of acupuncture. These systems have their own network and rules, which regulate their performance. It is already a familiar fact that we know so much today, yet still do not understand the energy system, though it is presumably derived from the metabolic pathways that are essential to life.

In order not to confuse the reader by charting overlapping systems on the feet, the diagrams show only the outline of the feet with its skeletal structure—without introducing the muscles, tendons, vessels, and meridians. The reflex zones have thus been represented in isolation, separate from their natural place in the living tissues that normally envelop them. However, this does make the method easier to learn.

In practice, the therapist will work on the reflexes of the nerve roots emerging from the lumbar and sacral segments of the spine (on the feet) without performing connective tissue massage and will encounter acupuncture points without doing acupuncture. Similarly, the periosteum of the bone will be probed without periosteal massage, and lymphatic reservoirs will be massaged without any actual practice of lymphatic drainage.

The similarity of shape between a sitting person and a foot also makes it easier to understand the location of the zones:

- The head and neck area is located in the toes.
- The chest area is in the middle of the foot.
- The stomach and loin area is at the base of the foot.

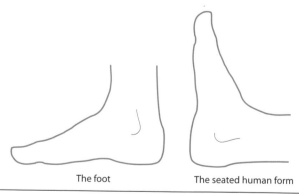

The foot   The seated human form

Figure 3. The flexed foot's shape is similar to that of a seated person.

Review of the
Reflex Zones of the Feet

It is frequently assumed that only the soles of the feet are important in reflex zone therapy, as they were more usually portrayed in the early pictures and diagrams. In fact, the whole foot—plantar and dorsal surfaces up to and including the inner and outer malleoli—should be included in a complete treatment. In general, the reflex zones of the organs can be readily palpated on the plantar aspect of the foot, while reflex zones of the bones, muscles, and nerves lie on the dorsal aspect.

The feet must be considered as a unity, and not as two separate entities. The entire portrait of the body can be seen true to scale in the feet, bearing in mind that it is primarily the head, neck, and trunk that are being mirrored. The treatment of the extremities developed more slowly over time.

Figure 4 summarizes the reflex zone system: every organ and tissue will generally find a corresponding reflex zone in the feet, lying in the same zone of the feet as in the body. The three cross sections of the body and the foot help practitioners to orient themselves. In addition, we can then use the correspondences shown in figures 5a–5d (pages 18–21) to see that:

- The organs of the right side of the body are found on the right foot, and the organs of the left side of the body are found on the left foot.

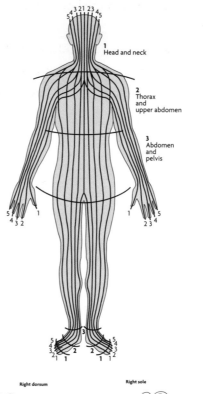

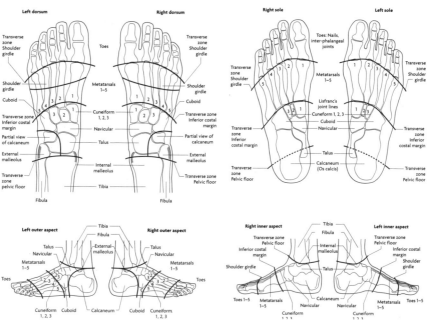

Figure 4. A summary of the reflex zone model system

- Organs that are paired in the body are found in paired zones on the left and right feet.
- Single organs are found once only, on either the left or right foot, depending on their anatomical position.
- Organs at the center of the body are found on the medial aspects of both feet.

The actual reflex zones terminate at the level of the ankle joint. Experience has shown, however, that treating areas within a handbreadth above the ankle joint can have great therapeutic value. Here lie additional reflex zones affecting the muscles and nerves of the lower extremities, especially from the thighs to the knees. They used to be considered "indirect" zones but are today recognized as independent zones.

The reflex zones of the upper extremities—up to the elbow—can be felt on the fifth metatarsal bone of the foot, and, like the zones for the lower extremities, they connect to the muscular and nerve network. These, too, used to be considered "indirect" zones.

Because of the closely woven fabric of connective tissue on the plantar heel, it is usually left out of treatment, except in children and those with tender feet. There is no therapeutic disadvantage in this, for these zones—which are the reflex zones to the pelvic organs—can be as easily treated on the rim or on either side of the heel as far as the ankle joint. With this approach a less vigorous massage is necessary for proper treatment.

Some zones can differ in proportion from the size or shape of the actual organ. However, daily practical experience confirms that every therapy represents a dynamic process that extends to the surrounding tissue, so that the calming effect of the treatment remains assured.

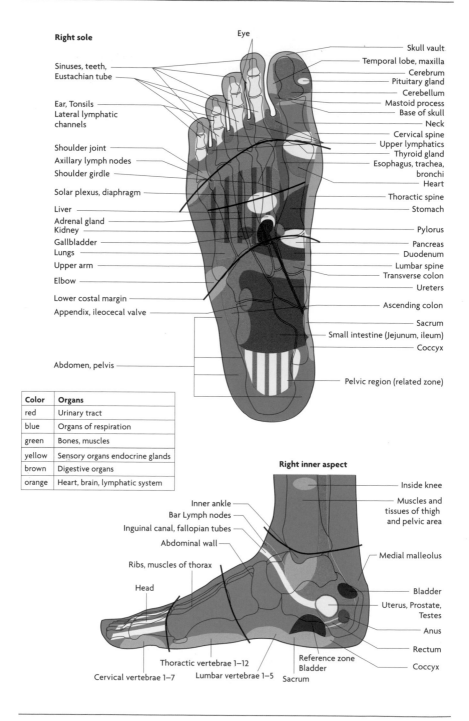

Right sole

Eye

Sinuses, teeth, Eustachian tube

Ear, Tonsils
Lateral lymphatic channels

Shoulder joint
Axillary lymph nodes
Shoulder girdle

Solar plexus, diaphragm

Liver
Adrenal gland
Kidney
Gallbladder
Lungs
Upper arm

Elbow

Lower costal margin
Appendix, ileocecal valve

Abdomen, pelvis

Skull vault
Temporal lobe, maxilla
Cerebrum
Pituitary gland
Cerebellum
Mastoid process
Base of skull
Neck
Cervical spine
Upper lymphatics
Thyroid gland
Esophagus, trachea, bronchi
Heart
Thoracic spine
Stomach
Pylorus
Pancreas
Duodenum
Lumbar spine
Transverse colon
Ureters
Ascending colon
Sacrum
Small intestine (Jejunum, ileum)
Coccyx
Pelvic region (related zone)

Color	Organs
red	Urinary tract
blue	Organs of respiration
green	Bones, muscles
yellow	Sensory organs endocrine glands
brown	Digestive organs
orange	Heart, brain, lymphatic system

Right inner aspect

Inside knee
Muscles and tissues of thigh and pelvic area

Inner ankle
Bar Lymph nodes
Inguinal canal, fallopian tubes
Abdominal wall

Medial malleolus

Ribs, muscles of thorax

Head

Bladder
Uterus, Prostate, Testes
Anus
Rectum
Coccyx

Thoracic vertebrae 1–12
Reference zone
Bladder

Cervical vertebrae 1–7   Lumbar vertebrae 1–5   Sacrum

Figure 5a. The microsystem of the feet mirrors
the macrosystem of the person.

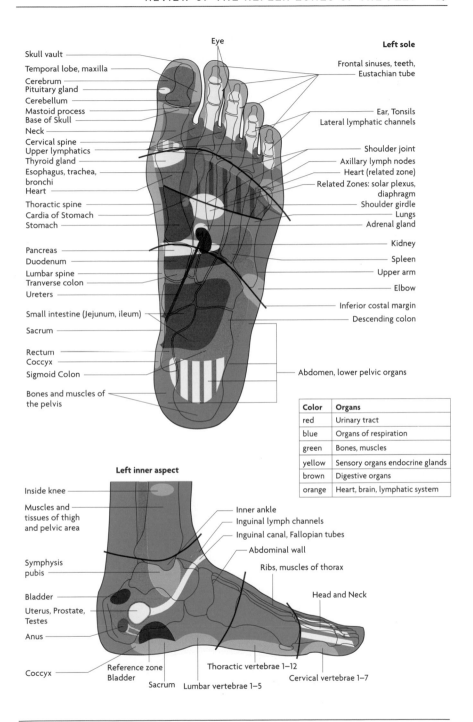

Figure 5b. The microsystem of the feet mirrors
the macrosystem of the person.

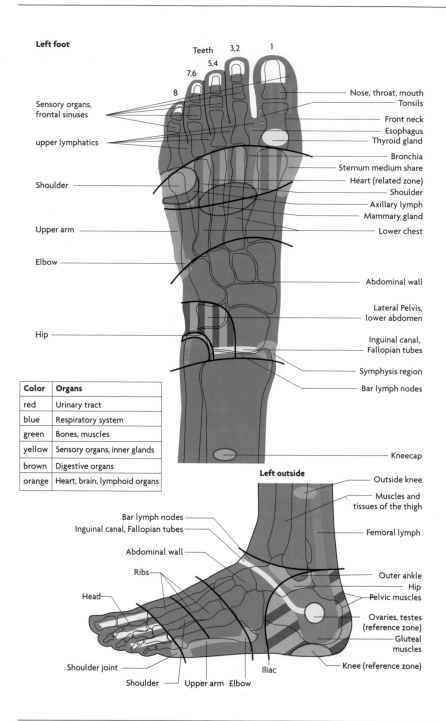

Left foot

Teeth   3,2   1
5,4
7,6
8

Nose, throat, mouth
Tonsils

Sensory organs, frontal sinuses

Front neck
Esophagus
Thyroid gland

upper lymphatics

Bronchia
Sternum medium share
Heart (related zone)
Shoulder
Axillary lymph
Mammary gland

Shoulder

Upper arm

Lower chest

Elbow

Abdominal wall

Lateral Pelvis, lower abdomen

Inguinal canal, Fallopian tubes

Hip

Symphysis region
Bar lymph nodes

Color	Organs
red	Urinary tract
blue	Respiratory system
green	Bones, muscles
yellow	Sensory organs, inner glands
brown	Digestive organs
orange	Heart, brain, lymphoid organs

Kneecap

Left outside

Outside knee
Muscles and tissues of the thigh

Bar lymph nodes
Inguinal canal, Fallopian tubes

Femoral lymph

Abdominal wall

Ribs

Outer ankle
Hip
Pelvic muscles

Head

Ovaries, testes (reference zone)
Gluteal muscles

Shoulder joint

Shoulder   Upper arm   Elbow   Iliac

Knee (reference zone)

Figure 5c. The microsystem of the feet mirrors
the macrosystem of the person.

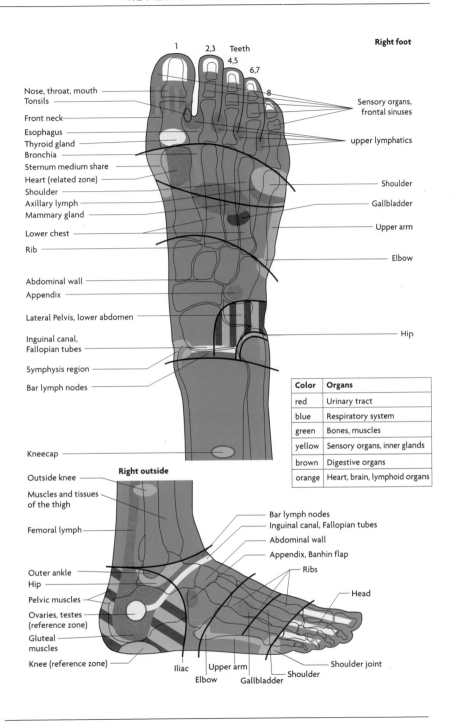

Right foot

1   2,3   Teeth
       4,5
              6,7
                 8

Nose, throat, mouth
Tonsils

Front neck

Esophagus
Thyroid gland
Bronchia
Sternum medium share
Heart (related zone)
Shoulder
Axillary lymph
Mammary gland

Lower chest

Rib

Abdominal wall
Appendix

Lateral Pelvis, lower abdomen

Inguinal canal,
Fallopian tubes

Symphysis region

Bar lymph nodes

Sensory organs,
frontal sinuses

upper lymphatics

Shoulder

Gallbladder

Upper arm

Elbow

Hip

Kneecap

Right outside

Outside knee
Muscles and tissues
of the thigh

Femoral lymph

Outer ankle
Hip
Pelvic muscles
Ovaries, testes
(reference zone)
Gluteal
muscles
Knee (reference zone)

Bar lymph nodes
Inguinal canal, Fallopian tubes
Abdominal wall
Appendix, Banhin flap
Ribs
Head

Iliac   Upper arm
    Elbow   Gallbladder   Shoulder

Shoulder joint

Color	Organs
red	Urinary tract
blue	Respiratory system
green	Bones, muscles
yellow	Sensory organs, inner glands
brown	Digestive organs
orange	Heart, brain, lymphoid organs

Figure 5d. The microsystem of the feet mirrors
the macrosystem of the person.

5

Burdened Reflex Zones of the Foot

We speak of reflex zones being burdened or distressed when they react with pain to treatment or when the autonomous nervous system produces signs of stress.

INDICATIONS OF BURDENED REFLEX ZONES ON THE FOOT

Some of the signs that a zone is overburdened include:

- Changes in a patient's expression
- Acoustic signals including sighing, groaning, whimpering, laughing, and so forth
- Gestures of pain, disquiet, or fear
- Visible contraction of different muscle groups, which may affect the whole body

Other, less obvious signs might be a spontaneous and perhaps profuse outbreak of sweat on the palms of the hands or over the whole body or changes in the patient's facial color, pulse rate, or saliva production.

INTERPRETATION OF THE BURDENED
REFLEX ZONES

Identifying a reflex zone that requires treatment allows the practitioner to draw conclusions about stress on the corresponding tissues or organ at the moment of treatment. It does not, however, allow for conclusions about the cause, type, or duration of the stress.

Distress in a given reflex zone may suggest:

1. Overtiredness, such as pain at the base of the spine after a long car journey
2. Overexertion—for example, strain on the heart after strenuous sport or a brain that is overtaxed after long hours of study
3. Latent disease whose symptoms have not yet become apparent
4. Acute disease processes, such as otitis media, gastritis, or nephritis
5. Chronic disease processes, such as chronic bronchitis, emphysema, tumors, or myocardial infirmity
6. Hyperactivity of an organ, for example hyperthyroidism
7. Hypoactivity of an organ, such as hypo- or achlorhydria of the stomach, or hormonal deficiencies
8. Palsy, atrophy, atony, or degeneration of an organ or tissue—as in a prolapsed uterus or rectum, floating kidneys, arthroses
9. Inherited predisposition to disease, which may include genetic tendencies toward skeletal or connective tissue weaknesses, allergies, or other inherited disorders
10. Previous accidents or injuries, such as fractures, sprains, or bruises

In the case of latent disease, the disturbed reflex zone may warn of such disease, and react abnormally in patients who are not as yet aware of illness. In such cases, reflex zones are found to be painful some days or even weeks before a noticeable symptom presents itself—such as an infection of the throat, or a painful limitation of the shoulder joint. It will be seen from the list above that the cause of an abnormal reflex zone is rarely a "crystalline deposit," as suggested by Ingham.[1] Such deposits will most likely occur among those suffering from rheumatism.

INTERPRETATION ATTEMPTS

In interpreting the causes of painful zones—whether they have appeared within seconds (as in the case of accidents) or have built up over many months (as in chronic illness)—we can draw on a wide range of practical experiences that have been extensively documented, as well as on a number of experimental studies.

We have, until now, considered the affected zones from the perspective of a functional energy failing: we recognize hyper-, hypo-, or a-tonus in the tissues of the feet, and speak in this context of an energy stream that is not physiological but is perceptible in the tissues as an energy fullness, an energy deficiency, or an energy absence. The autonomic nervous system in particular gives clear indications of the stress of individual zones (sweaty hands, dry mouth, changes in respiration, and so forth; see chapter 14).

For these reasons, the therapist will refrain from rash "diagnoses" that would only call into question his or her own credibility. Moreover, we have observed that in some severe psychological illnesses or terminal cancer cases (particularly when the patient is undergoing cobalt treatment), the reflex zones of the feet do not always give an exact picture of the physical condition of the patient at that time. It may also happen that infirmity of an organ is not perceived in a reflex zone only, but may even prefer to leave another "signature"—for example in the connective tissue or in the acupuncture meridians.

GENERAL CAUSES

A number of external and internal causes can lead to stress on the foot. If and when one of these causes leads to distressed reflex zones depends on the duration and intensity of the cause as well as the vitality of the person. Situations that can lead to foot pain include:

- Over exertion: extreme hiking, running, one-sided sports
- Fatigue and exhaustion, including those occupations that necessitate standing all day, especially on concrete floors
- Acute injuries, such as wounds, cuts, perforating or penetrating foreign objects, stings, fractures, and sprains
- Inherited conditions, such as weakness of the connective tissue; flat feet or splay feet; valgus or varux toes
- General circulatory disturbances, such as varicose veins, varicose ulcers, ulcus cruris, Buerger's disease, intermittent claudication, and so forth
- Rheumatoid disease, widespread or localized, which may manifest itself in the feet, for example with arthritic toes

Even when foot problems are not directly related to stress on their respective zones, problems of the feet always affect and weaken a person's overall well-being.

6

Symptomatic and Background Zones

Symptomatic zones are the areas on the foot that relate directly to the symptoms exhibited by the patient. In a patient with gastritis, for example, this is the stomach zone; in a patient with a shoulder injury, the shoulder zone.

The *background zones* (formerly called *causal reflex zones*) refer to the reflex zones of the foot that mark the background of a condition, or the area where the patient's reported ailments originated. In a patient with headache this could be the zone of the liver, intestine, or spine, or in the case of a woman with painful menstruation, the zone of the pelvis.

It is not necessary to treat all theoretically possible background zones for every disease picture. Selection of individual zones depends on the visual and palpable observations made on the feet of each patient (see initial assessment, pages 48–49). When a reflex zone is abnormal (resulting in pain, sweaty hands, and so forth) it is treated, otherwise not.

From this maxim follows the fundamental principle that every patient should have every reflex zone tested for sensitivity, and practitioners should perform both visual and palpatory examinations during the first reflex zone massage. This is the only way for a therapist to build an objective picture of the initial presenting condition of the patient. This initial exam then serves as a guideline for the whole subsequent series of treatments. Therapy will vary in successive treatments according to the patient's account of the nature, duration, and severity of the reactions that have taken place since the previous treatment.

Exceptions to the notion of full-zone exams are first-aid treatments or, those for acute ailments, where we confine treatment solely to the symptomatic zone as well as a selection of directly relevant background zones (see acute treatment, page 40).

7

Indications for Therapists and Laypeople

Reflex zone therapy of the feet has a broad range of good uses, but it is also important to note its limitations. In particular, it is helpful—especially for laypeople—to distinguish between *treating illness* and *maintaining health*.

The treatment of illness should be done only by medical/therapeutic professionals, for example doctors, physical therapists, psychotherapists, licensed massage therapists, nurses, podiatrists, and so forth. People who are not part of the medical profession can work under the guidance of a doctor or healing practitioner, but they should not attempt to treat serious illnesses on their own.

At the same time, it is as important as ever to maintain health, meaning that there is much room for treatments by nonprofessionals. They can work within their family and circle of friends, but should limit themselves to treating healthy people with short-term minor ailments.

Whether you are a medical professional or an interested layperson, you can benefit many people with reflex zone therapy. Being touched is a basic human need that almost everyone responds to, including children and older adults.

INDICATIONS FOR MEDICAL PROFESSIONALS

Uses of reflex zone therapy include:

- Acute and chronic tendinomuscular ailments, including spinal problems, lumbar strains, arthrosis, pain and movement limitations of the shoulder and pelvic girdles
- Functional disturbances of the digestive system such as gastritis, acid reflux, chronic constipation, diarrhea, problems in the gall flow, hemorrhoids
- Strain on the respiratory system, including chronic illnesses, bronchitis, acute cough
- Ailments of the urinary tract such as cystitis (without fever), insufficient or excessive urination
- Allergies such as hay fever, bronchial asthma, skin problems, and food allergies
- Chronic sleep problems with organic and/or emotional causes, such as dietary issues or traumatic events
- Functional disturbances of the female pelvic organs, for example very light or heavy menstruation, or strong pain or mood swings before, during, or after menstruation

INDICATIONS FOR NONPROFESSIONAL HEALERS

Anyone who wants to treat the feet of others can do so as long as they do not claim to be healing illnesses. Some everyday ailments that respond well to episodic treatment include:

- Tendinomuscular pains of the back, shoulders, or knees, as may occur after long car rides, exertion in the garden, or intensive sports, for example
- Digestive problems—such as flatulence after a meal, constipation

following change of place or climate, or diarrhea following sudden excitement

- Susceptibility to colds, temporarily dry mucous membranes
- Frequent urination during emotional stress
- Menstrual cramping, light pelvic pain following a birth
- Temporary sleep problems
- Emotional changes, for example those caused by stress at work or home

8

Contraindications

As with all therapies, reflex zone therapy of the feet has its limits, beyond which its practice is ineffective. Contraindications to therapy are:

- Acute infectious fevers and diseases
- Deep vein thrombosis and acute inflammations of the venous or lymphatic systems
- Conditions where surgery is indicated
- Complex regional pain syndrome (CRPS) that affects the feet
- Gangrene and extensive fungal infections of the feet
- Pregnancies that are unstable or at risk
- Osteoporosis and decalcification resulting from poor healing or nonunion of bone; possible decalcification resulting from tumors

Experience has shown that, apart from the conditions listed above, chronic and progressive or terminal illnesses (such as ankylosing spondylitis, multiple sclerosis, Parkinson's disease, cancer, and paralysis) will often respond to treatment of the reflex zones of the feet. The disease may not be amenable to cure, but the patient may often be made more comfortable. The following improvements may accompany treatment:

- Functional improvement of the organs of excretion—the kidneys, intestines, skin, and lungs
- Alleviation of pain, even in the terminal stages of cancer and during renal dialysis
- Increase in control of the sphincter muscles of the bladder and bowels

Patients whose recent surgery has resulted in retention of urine may frequently be spared catheterization if the reflex zones of the bladder and solar plexus are treated. Such noninvasive treatment is already being successfully carried out in some hospitals in Europe.

PART TWO

PRACTICAL
APPLICATION

9

Positioning
the Patient

The correct positioning of the patient is an important preparation for reflex zone massage of the feet and will facilitate your work. This includes:

- A well-ventilated, warm, and well-lit room, with adequate space for patient and therapist
- A wide, well-upholstered couch or massage table
- No disturbing background noise
- Cushions for head, neck, and knees should be used as necessary
- A light blanket (preferably not of synthetic fabric) should be used to cover the patient, as some loss of body heat accompanies each massage. In addition, most patients find it easier to relax in an atmosphere of personal attention when they're covered. Lastly, patients who are covered will be less shy of allowing their legs to relax and fall into the necessary outwardly rotated position.

When the patient is lying down comfortably, he or she should loosen any constricting clothing (belt, brassiere, corset, collar, tie, trousers) so that he or she may breathe easily and freely.

The patient should lie in a supine position with the head slightly raised. This enables the therapist to constantly observe the facial expres-

sion and any spontaneous reaction—whether of pain or relaxation—
and consequently adjust the massage appropriately. From this position
the patient may also view the therapist at work. This is of the greatest
importance at the start of treatment in order to build up a relationship
of trust.

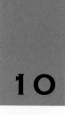

10

The Grip Sequence

People have become accustomed nowadays to the idea that a "technique" is necessary to the performance of any therapy, and we often speak of "breathing techniques," "movement techniques," "massage techniques," and so forth. The use of this word can be restrictive, however, and for our purpose is better avoided, for *technique* can imply solely the mechanical and the material, and implicit in its use is a limitation to these two domains.

Human beings inhabit three dimensions, even in their locomotion. Because of the existence of joints, movements are fluid and curved—not stiff and angular—when the original upright posture is maintained. Unfortunately, it is still possible to move in a two-dimensional and restricted manner. The fluidity of movement is then lost, muscles become overstretched and misaligned, and the flowing dynamic coordination of each part becomes obstructed. This can be true of small as well as large joints.

Therefore, to start with, the hands of the therapist must be rightly positioned. Whether at rest or in the working position, the hand should hold the foot in a natural, loose, and relaxed position, without overstretching the muscles or rigidly fixing the joints. A healthy distance to the feet of the patient is about the length of the practitioner's forearm.

The thumb adopts a special position facing the fingers. Because of its greater strength, and because it has a greater radius of movement from its base joint, the thumb is preferred during treatment, especially for beginners. Because of the thumb's great flexibility, the therapist is able to encircle the foot of the patient and literally take it into his hands. When working on the sole of the foot with the thumb, the fingers support the dorsum of the foot and vice versa. For the back of the foot, however, it is better to use the index finger.

There are four steps to each grip:

1. The touch is the first step and one often not given enough attention. The quality of the touch determines whether a relationship of trust can be built between therapist and patient. The touch should be attentive, gentle, and clear.

2. With the second step, the active phase begins. This phase does not begin with the working finger (which would cause mechanical pressure), but rather with an active gentle forward swing of the bent arm. This allows the joint of the thumb or working finger to reach the foot at an 80–90 degree angle with hardly any effort of its own.

3. Only when this forward swing reaches its maximum is deliberate pressure applied by the thumb or forefinger to the tissues of the foot. This is the third step.

4. From this activity flows the fourth step, when the thumb is allowed to return passively from the tissue depths to its original position on the skin surface and resume the slack resting position of the passive stage. This also marks the beginning of the next sequence.

Continually alternating these active and passive phases, the thumb proceeds millimeter by millimeter across the surface of the skin and the underlying reflex zones, giving rise to an undulating rhythm and a flowing energy distribution in the painful tissues of the feet.

The thumb should always move forward, and never lose contact with the surface of the skin during the treatment sequence. If the therapist attempts to move the thumb backward, that is, toward his own body rather than away from it, the smooth flowing movement becomes disjointed and impeded. Whether a reflex zone is treated from left to right or from heel to toe is of secondary importance; the approach is dictated by the state of tissue tonus or the best positioning of the hand.

When the thumb of the therapist is kinked to a right angle, the movement is incorrect, as the forward flowing movement becomes rigid and angular and the thumbnails come into contact with the skin surface, giving rise to unnecessary pain. Furthermore, this position leads to a mechanical pressure, which tires the therapist more rapidly and thus makes it impossible to fully exploit the possibilities of regenerating the patient's tissue.

To better understand the special therapeutic touch, the differences between physiologically correct and mechanical, exhausting grips are reviewed once more below:

- A movement that causes the end of the thumb or index finger to enter the tissue at a right angle exhausts therapist as well as patient, because it is mechanical and applied with pressure.
- In contrast, organic physiological work depends on concepts like strength, dynamic movement, rhythm, feeling, and flow. It may be helpful to picture a child bouncing a ball and observe how the ball bounces upward after touching the ground.

Even when the thumbnail does not make contact with the tissues of the feet, the sharp, prickling pain of disturbed reflex zones will frequently give rise to a mistaken belief in the patient's mind that it is the therapist's nails that are the cause, for he will often be unable to distinguish between the injury from the outside and the sensation of pain in his own tissues. When this happens, it is essential that the patient can trust the explanation of the therapist, that he has a sense of being correctly treated, and that pressure is reduced.

In skilled and experienced hands, the grip sequence can be altered. Thoughtful modifications can transform the procedure from a slow progress across the individual reflex zones of the feet into a vital therapy of the disordered systems of the body. This potential is what gives reflex zone therapy its validity as a therapy. This is so even when the patient suffers severe impairment of the tissues owing to disease or injury in more than one system and treatment must be carefully integrated. There are similar developmental parallels in other methods, when treatment must be graduated and modified according to circumstances. Even Vicar Kneipp (a famous pastor in Germany who invented a specific form of cold water therapy) recounted that he "had to put aside my earlier drastic applications . . . and I was converted from great mildness to even greater mildness in my cures."[1]

The neutral grip sequence described above can be enhanced in two ways:

1. By varying the working *rhythm* and *tempo*
2. By varying the *intensity,* which depends on the amount of energy expended

These options allow the practitioner to choose between two general styles: slow and deliberate work, which has calming effects, and swift, uninterrupted work. This style is strong and reaches deep into the tissue, producing an energizing effect. Do not think, however, that the hand has only muscular strength to deliver; it has the resources to work effectively with dexterity, and a delicate strength that is not bound to visible muscular power.

There is no fixed rule for determining what should be the intensity and what the expenditure of energy in any given treatment. No two people react in the same way, and one person will react differently to the same stimulus as his internal and external circumstances alter. In general, the therapist works up to the individual patient's pain threshold, and only then, when the pain diminishes and is overcome, can tissue turgor begin to return to normal.

Neither can there be any rigid dictates as to the duration of each grip sequence, that is, the length of time that pressure is exerted during the active phase. In earlier times, practitioners sometimes relied on painful stimuli for several minutes at a time; today a second-long impulse frequently suffices to bring about a regenerative effect. These second-long impulses may be repeated several times during a reflex zone massage in order to bring the tissues into a healthier state of tonus.

If the patient is in great pain, much debilitated, or overwrought, even careful pressure on a reflex zone may breach the pain threshold. This is more likely to happen when the patient is in a weakened nervous state (whether this is temporary or of long standing is beside the point) or when an organ is in an acute reactive phase. Pay very careful attention here, and use just that degree of pressure that calms and restores the patient. Frequently and gently stretch and stroke the feet and legs.

Once the fingers have become more receptive, they can also execute fine vibratory and stretching movements on appropriate areas of the feet. The swinging elasticity of the fingertips in such grips, and their rhythmical intrusion into the tissues of feet can produce profound effects.

THE SEDATION GRIP

When treating patients with acute pain (colic, acute earache, neuralgia, hemorrhoids, injuries, toothache, and so forth), the movement is so adapted that it alleviates pain and calms the patient. This is accomplished by using a firm hold that is sustained for 30–60 seconds while fingers and thumbs maintain an even pressure on the painful tissues. In this way, we move slowly from the surface of the tissue into its depth, paying close attention to the facial expressions of the patient since it helps us find the right dose. It often happens that the pain in an organ subsides or disappears within a short time: 10–20 seconds. Just as the tension is reduced in the reflex zone, pain in the respective organ or joint often improves as well.

This sedation grip may be used as a form of first-aid, though the fact that you may need to use it during a treatment does not exclude the possibility of your continuing to treat other organs and systems in order to seek out the underlying cause of the patient's condition (working, of course, within the limits of the patient's tolerance).

Efforts to have a balanced grip on the foot should not hide the fact that not every detail of every zone or symptom is essential for the therapy. Rather, a holistic approach to the person will dictate what zones and symptoms to focus on.

Finally, I should note that no amount of written description can replace the practical experience gained through patient practice.

11

The First Treatment

The first treatment is the most important opportunity to evaluate the overall condition of the patient, and the specific condition of the feet. Physical treatment should begin only after thorough examinations have been made and a diagnosis has been reached.

FINDING A DIAGNOSIS

The patient's feet should lie within easy reach of the practitioner, who should be relaxed and seated with spine erect. The distance between the feet of the patient and the practitioner will be dictated by the length of the practitioner's loosely flexed arms. This maintains a healthy distance. The patient's feet rest on the massage table and must not be supported on the knees or thighs of the therapist. The manner of working must be so relaxed and flexible that if at any time during the treatment the patient wishes to withdraw his feet, he may do so and does not feel that he must helplessly endure the pain. He is likely, otherwise, to become anxious, cramped, tense, or angry.

True pain will disturb the patient less when she is able to breathe easily and freely, and when she opens herself up as much as possible to the therapy. This also enables her to follow the massage procedure with attention and interest and not to believe that her attention should be diverted through chatter or by misdirected concentration or relaxation exercises. She can, if she wishes, be wholly attentive to events at the site of therapy as they are being experienced in her feet.

Visual Evaluation

Visual evaluation takes place before the touch evaluation. By itself it does not give objective conclusions on the patient's condition, but serves as a complement to later evaluation by touch. At the end of the first treatment, its findings are indicated on the patient chart in pencil.

Beginners will at first have a hard time observing the total surfaces of the feet; they must have patience and learn first to palpate and observe the smaller surface areas of the feet. It will soon be appreciated that although every foot has the same basic anatomical structure, each bears entirely personal and noteworthy characteristics. For this reason, working with the feet is never boring or monotonous; the therapist approaches with interest the individual picture of the person engraved on their feet, and perceives the result of his endeavors in the reactions that follow.

Any departure from the normal color, shape, tissue turgor, or temperature evident in the feet and persisting for longer than a few weeks may be the external expression of a disturbed reflex zone. Visual examination includes the following:

1. The bony structure
2. The condition of the tissues
3. The condition of the skin and nails

Visual Examination of the Bony Structure of the Feet

The importance of the feet as arched structures that bear the weight of the whole body is well known and important to the practice of many other physical therapy disciplines, including orthopedics and chiropracty. They view the foot principally from the perspective of its dynamic equilibrium. This approach, although different, complements and enhances our knowledge of the feet when we practice reflex zone therapy.

Changes in the skeletal structure of the feet mean that there is a disturbance in the energy distribution in the reflex zones. It follows that there is a relationship between any alteration of the normal alignment of the bony structure of the feet and a disorder in corresponding organs of the body.

For example,

- A flattened, splayed transverse arch can affect the reflex zone of the shoulder girdle and organs of respiration, and/or the liver and gallbladder on the right foot, or the heart on the left.
- Fallen arches or flat feet can affect the reflex zones of the spinal column.
- Hallux valgus has its effect upon the reflex zones of the cervical spine and the thyroid gland.
- Hammertoe and other deformities of the toes burden all the reflex zones of the head and the teeth.
- Fungally infected toenails (onychomycosis) or nails that are noticeably abnormal in shape and texture (wooden nails) indicate that the reflex zones of the head have been in some way affected.
- Injury or congestion on the heel or around the inner and outer malleoli are associated with disorders of the pelvis and hip joints.
- Sunken cuneiform bones imply disease of the intestine.

Visual Examination of the Tissues

The feet show lymphatic congestion and edema (pitting edema) primarily in the region of the ankle, around the malleoli, at the Achilles tendon, and above the bases of the toe joints on the dorsum of the feet. These are the reflex zones of the pelvis and the organs of the upper thorax.

Edema around the malleoli may in general be attributed to a disorder of the kidneys, heart, or circulation. We have also found patients with this symptom to have considerable congestion in the pelvis, which may be of venous, arterial, lymphatic, nervous system, or hormonal origin. There is without doubt an associated disturbance of circulation, but this is secondary.

Diseases of the heart and circulation are frequently evident to the therapist making a visual examination; they appear as tiny pads around the base of the toes on the left dorsum.

Visual Examination of the Skin

The skin of most people's feet is rough and neglected. It is therefore an excellent source of information when visually examined. The type of abnormality or deformity on the foot is not particularly relevant, what is far more important is its site.

For example, a corn at the metatarso-phalangeal joint of the small toe on the left foot reflects some injury to the shoulder. A corn between the right second and third toes bears on the reflex zone of the right eye. Whether it's a corn, a callous, or a mycotic infection like athlete's foot that appears over the reflex zone, what is important is the visible alteration in the condition of the skin, which thereby indicates that the corresponding reflex zone may be affected.

The skin of the feet should be examined for the following abnormalities: cracks and crevices; warts and fissures in the webs between the toes; dull, cold, or throbbing skin; athlete's foot; wounds, corns, or blisters; heat rash, varicose veins, or odor; pigmentation, reddening, desquamation, sweating of the feet, pustules, pimples, vesicles, ulcers; horniness, indentations, puffiness, scars; the shape, color, and texture of each individual toenail.

> **Note:** Varicose veins that lie in the vicinity of any of the reflex zones, that is to say on the lower third of the leg between the knee and ankle joints, should be avoided during reflex zone massage. The same is true for ulcers in this area.

Although a variety of different external factors—like tight shoes, socks, or stockings, athlete's foot, fashionably high but unhealthy shoes, footwear made of unsuitable materials, or inadequate personal hygiene— may account for such abnormalities, they are not often the true cause.

The ailments frequently encounter a favorable milieu for their development because of some inherent weakness or predisposition to weakness in the reflex zone over which they appear. In other words, an internal debilitation is present in many cases before the external disorder arises.

For example, athlete's foot rarely extends over the entire foot, and does not often even affect all the webs between the toes if one has been exposed to infection at a swimming pool or sauna bath. It is typically observed in a specific site, which nearly always coincides with overtaxation of the related organ. A sound and healthy foot would rapidly overcome infection by local application of fungicides or by careful attention to the area. Only when the underlying reflex zone is disordered will such infections thrive.

Even though the patient does not complain—and may not be aware—of dysfunction of an organ or system in his body, this does not mean the absence of disease. He believes, erroneously, that the absence of pain and lack of awareness of the disordered function of his own body is synonymous with health. Athlete's foot is often highly resistant to any form of external treatment and only heals completely when local external treatment gives rise to a changed and restored internal condition.

Reflex zone massage of the feet is appropriate to bringing about this restoration. With repeated treatments, the circulation to this affected area of skin improves. This decreases the perimeter in which the microorganisms can flourish.

Note: Therapy is not carried out on areas infected by any fungus. Instead, it is directed from healthy tissues toward the diseased parts, but only as far as is hygienically acceptable for the therapist and tolerable for the patient.

A chiropodist or podiatrist, who must complete an intensive training, is an invaluable colleague for the therapist, particularly when he or she has learned and assimilated the principles of reflex zone therapy. A podiatrist will treat the feet sensitively and will maintain them in the best possible condition. To this end, corns and calluses are pared away, nails are cut and shaped, and ingrown toenails are prevented.

Because the visual examination is so important, and the source of so much information for the therapist, it is preferable for the patient to visit the podiatrist after the first reflex zone massage rather than beforehand.

Touch Evaluation

The therapist establishes contact by taking the feet in her hands and at the same time making a few gentle stroking movements. This provides her with a neutral first impression of the condition of the patient and the temperature of the feet.

During the massage, both hands should always be on the foot. While one hand works, the other supports and maintains contact. (With much experience and practice, the grip sequence can be used bimanually, in which case all the fingers will be used in massage. The practical application and exact methods for such variations must be gained through instruction courses, since the experience of palpation cannot be theoretically transmitted.)

Correct pressure during palpation will yield the most fruitful results. To assess the correct pressure, note the spontaneous reactions of the patient to your first impulse of pressure. If the patient jerks her foot backward or makes an involuntary expression of pain, the intensity of your massage must be immediately reduced. If the patient is calm and still, or has the sensation of being lightly tickled, her individual pain threshold has not been reached.

When you have found the appropriate intensity of your massage grip sequence—one that the patient finds bearable—you should maintain this level of intensity for the duration of the first treatment. It is best to include parts of the foot that are known to be burdened among many people—the zones of the lower spine, the neck, or the intestines. Since the same dosage on different parts of the foot will elicit different reactions, this allows a way to compare healthy tissue with zones that require treatment.

In a set sequence, all zones are briefly checked for ailments (pain, vegetative signs). The zones in need of treatment are then colored onto the treatment map together with a short summary (see figure 6). This map allows the therapist to quickly recall the symptomatic zones as well as their

Patient chart for reflex zone therapy on the foot

Patient information: _____

Name: _____ Gender/Age: _____

Patient symptoms (or diagnosis from sending doctor if referral) _____

_____

Medications currently taken: _____

Other treatments: _____

Medical history: illnesses, surgeries, accidents, scars: _____

_____

Teeth: fillings (type), root treatments _____

_____

For initial assessment:
Color symptomatic zones red, background zones green, visual findings black

Intensity of the zones:
Very intense: shade deeply, medium: medium, little: light

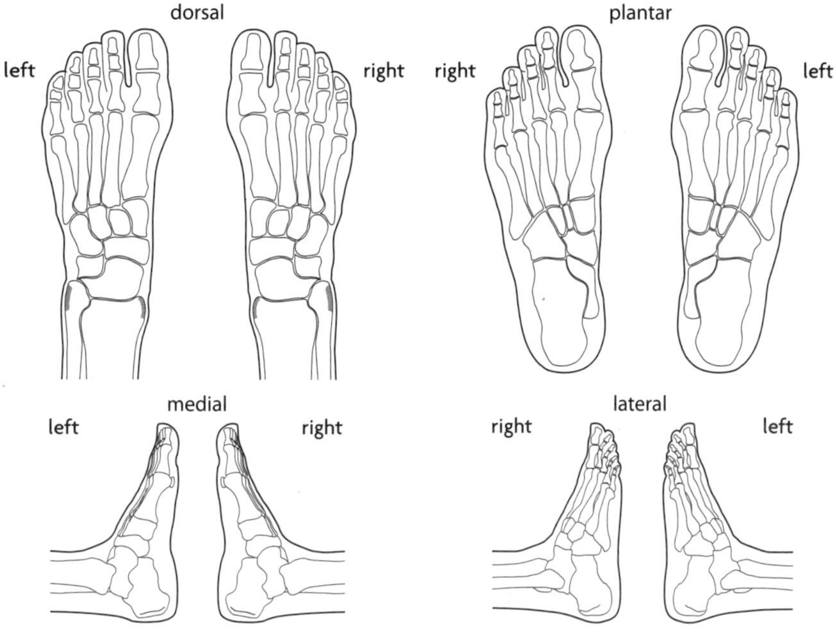

dorsal

left   right   right   left

plantar

medial

left   right   right   left

lateral

Figure 6. Example of a blank patient chart

Applications:

Date	Reactions during application	Reactions between applications

Final result:
After how many treatments did the condition change noteably? _____

What symptoms have changes?
From point of view of therapist (objective): _____

From point of view of patient (subjective): _____

Other observations and notes
(for example reduced consumption _____
of medication, weight changes, etc):

Figure 6. Example of a blank patient chart, continued

backgrounds each time that patient visits. This thorough and objective testing of the zones offers the opportunity to let go of preconceived symptoms and to recognize the person as a whole.

The first reflex zone massage of the feet usually takes about 50–60 minutes. Subsequent treatments are usually shorter—25–30 minutes—since only those zones that require treatment are covered. Although the first observation of the zones can cause reactions, it does not represent the actual therapy; only subsequent treatments stabilize the therapeutic effect.

Treatment is most effective when the second-long pressure impulse is repeated at frequent intervals, not continuously, to the same area during a reflex zone massage. On this point in particular the past decades have seen significant changes. The treatment intervals lasting several minutes at a time that were used in the past would not be bearable for many patients today. With each repetition of the second-long pressure impulse, the area will be less painful, which will be due in part to the improvement in circulation that follows massage.

Treatment is complete when the intense local pain in the disturbed reflex zones decreases to a level that is bearable for the patient. This usually happens within 20–30 minutes, but there will always be exceptions, and one patient may require only 15 minutes and another up to 50 minutes before the tissue tonus begins to be restored to normal.

People react differently to the same therapeutic stimulus, according to their own personal disease backgrounds. It is also true that the same person will respond differently to the same therapy from time to time because of any of a number of changes that may have occurred in the inner and outer environment, such as:

- Change of climate
- Active or passive phase of personal biorhythms
- Change of diet
- Emotional state
- Early, and as yet unremarked, stages of many illnesses
- Commencement of the reaction stage and healing crisis

12

Treatment Sequence

The following sequence has proven effective in practice, especially for those new to this type of therapy.

ZONES OF HEAD AND NECK

The reflex zones of the head display a marked peculiarity. While they are distributed over all ten toes, they are further replicated in miniature on both large toes. For this reason, treatment of the head zones begins on the two big toes (see figure 7 on page 53).

Rotation of the big toe around the metatarso-phalangeal joint is the reflex equivalent of rotating the atlas on the axis (that is, rotating the head on the neck). Any minute deposits that are present may make themselves heard or felt during such rotation through pain, crackling, friction, or by limitation of movement; all of these reactions point to a corresponding disorder in the region of the head and/or neck. To double-check this, the patient can sit down and compare the correspondence of the burdens in the neck area with the range of motion of the base joints of the big toes.

The areas corresponding to the nose, mouth, and throat occupy a relatively large area on the dorsum of the big toe, while the surrounding tissues represent the bones and musculature of the face.

The pad of the big toe represents the posterior aspect of the head, while its dorsal surface bears the reflex zones that represent the face. The transverse crease that marks the proximal boundary of the pad of the big toe is the reflex zone that accords with the base of the skull.

When these areas have been treated on the big toes, the reflex zones of these same structures are then treated on the individual toes, where they are found in larger scale. Those reflex zones that correspond to the eyes and ears are best approached from the soles, while the sinuses and teeth may be treated from both plantar and dorsal aspects.

The teeth of the upper jaw are found between the distal and middle creases of the joints of the toes, while the teeth of the lower jaw are located on the dorsum around the middle and dorsal joint creases.

The reflex zones of the teeth are also exactly distributed over the ten zones spanning the toes, and are arranged as follows:

Incisors	(1)	Body zone 1	Big toe
Incisors and canine teeth	(2, 3)	Body zone 2	Second toe
Premolars	(4, 5)	Body zone 3	Third toe
Molars	(6, 7)	Body zone 4	Fourth toe
Wisdom teeth	(8)	Body zone 5	Fifth toe

Note: During treatment, both medial and lateral sides of the toes are naturally included, even though they are not shown on the diagrams.

The tissue forming the webs of the toes reflects the upper lymphatic system, and a good blood supply to these areas is achieved by taking them in a pincer grasp and drawing them firmly toward you, while gently flexing the ball of the foot at the same time. (This movement is similar to that used when milking a cow!) In the interests of hygiene, and in order not to spread infection, these areas are not treated on people with athlete's foot or other fungal infections until the infection has been cured.

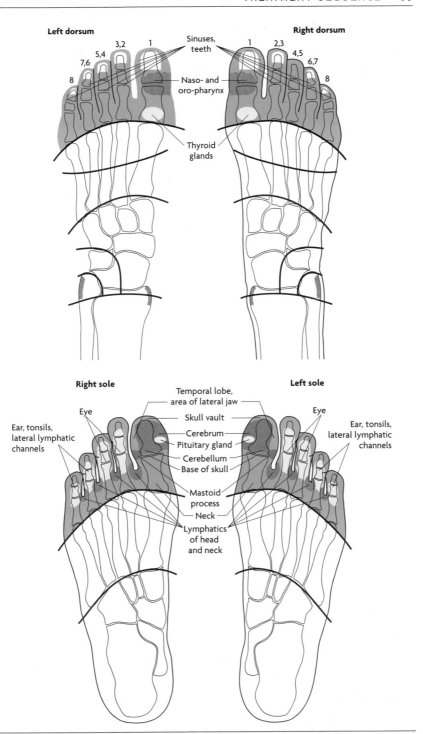

Figure 7. Reflex zones of the head

ZONES OF THE
MUSCULOSKELETAL SYSTEM

The reflex zones of the spine, joints, and muscles are described below and can be seen in figures 8a and 8b (pages 56–57).

Spinal Column

The reflex zones of the spinal column are situated along the longitudinal arches on the medial aspects of both feet.

- The zones of the cervical spine are found along the entire length of the proximal phalanx of each big toe, beginning just a little distally to the interphalangeal joint, which is the reflex zone of the base of the skull.
- The zones of the thoracic (or dorsal) spine are found along the medial aspect of the first metatarsal bone on both feet.
- The zones of the lumbar spine are found along the medial aspect of the first cuneiform bone and the distal half of the scaphoid bone.
- The zones of the sacrum begin at the proximal part of the scaphoid bone and continue along part of the talus.
- The zones of the coccyx are found along the distal third of the calcaneum.

These reflex zones are usually not massaged by applying pressure to the periosteum, but rather by attention to the muscles that clothe them, slightly toward the sole.

The joint formed by the phalanx of the big toe and the first metatarsal bone, which is the reflex zone of the lower cervical and upper thoracic spine, requires careful observation. This joint often shows pathological changes in the form of a hallux valgus (lateral flexion of the big toe). Due to the altered alignment of the bones in this condition, the reflex zones of the neck will be affected. It is often not possible to clearly identify the primary and secondary connections here; usually this is a dynamic relationship between foot and neck.

Note: Reflex zone massage before treatment by a chiropractor, osteopath, or manual therapist has proven to be useful. Intense muscular spasm treated by reflex zone massage preparatory to manipulation of the vertebrae ensures that the procedure is less painful to the patient and requires less energetic manipulation. From time to time muscles and tendons that have been relaxed in this way permit a vertebra to slip back into position (usually a cervical vertebra) during reflex zone massage to the feet. In this case, the patient may hear and feel the vertebra returning to its normal position.

Observation of hundreds of patients has shown that when a hallux valgus is present, there are nearly always concomitant symptoms, including tension of the neck and shoulder muscles, spinal problems, and/or dysfunction of the thyroid gland or heart.

The physical distortion of bone and muscle structures, and the subsequent effects on the skeletal, postural, and supporting systems, forms a pathological picture that has been supplemented by the empirical experience of reflex zone massage.

Reflex Zones of the Neck and Shoulders

The zones of the neck are located on the plantar part of the base joint of the big toes. The zones of the shoulder girdle are found on both plantar and dorsal aspects, spanning the transverse arches formed by the distal halves of the metatarsal bones. On the plantar surface, work on the reflex zone of the right shoulder will also indirectly treat the reflex zones of the liver and gallbladder (because of their related segmental innervation). By the same token, work on the plantar reflex zone of the left shoulder girdle will simultaneously stimulate the reflex zone of the heart.

The dorsal reflex zone of the shoulder girdle has long been recognized. It overlies the distal half of all five metatarsal bones (as described above), and should be included in all treatment of the shoulder girdle, corresponding as it does to the ventral surface of the thorax. Experience has shown that once tension in the interstices between the metatarsal bones

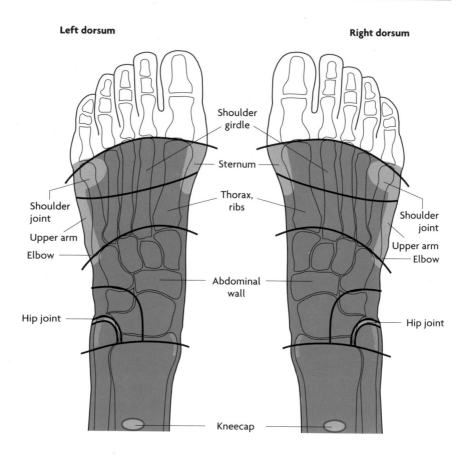

Left dorsum

Right dorsum

Shoulder
girdle

Sternum

Shoulder
joint

Thorax,
ribs

Shoulder
joint

Upper arm

Upper arm

Elbow

Elbow

Abdominal
wall

Hip joint

Hip joint

Kneecap

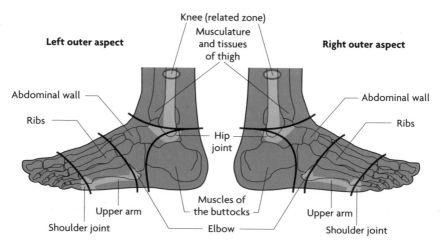

Knee (related zone)

Musculature
and tissues
of thigh

Left outer aspect

Right outer aspect

Abdominal wall

Abdominal wall

Ribs

Ribs

Hip
joint

Upper arm

Upper arm

Shoulder joint

Muscles of
the buttocks

Shoulder joint

Elbow

Figure 8a. Zones of the spine, joints, and muscles of the body

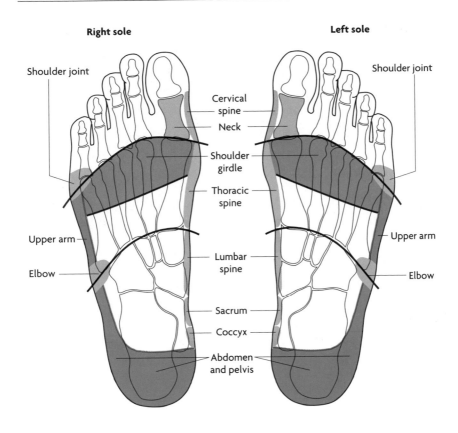

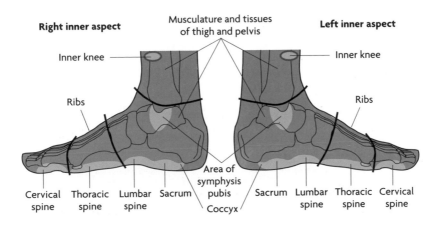

Figure 8b. Zones of the spine, joints, and muscles of the body

on the dorsum of the feet has been alleviated, the musculature and nerve tracts of the shoulder girdle can be more competently treated.

> **Note:** A special relationship has been found in the shoulder girdle zones between physical and mental symptoms. Muscular rigidity and decreased flexibility of the transverse arches betoken not only a physical disorder, but also the burdens of psychic stress that people "carry on their shoulders."

The reflex zone that corresponds to the shoulder joint is easily recognized in the feet, mirrored in the articulation of each small toe with the fifth metatarsal bone. Note that the lateral borders of the fifth metatarsal bones are, on the one hand the reflex zones of the lateral aspect of the thorax and on the other hand are also zones of the upper arm as far as the elbow joint, which lies at the base of the fifth metatarsal bone.

The reflex zone of the sternum is situated on the distal dorsal surface to the left and right of the first metatarsal bone. There is a relationship between this zone and those of the heart, organs of respiration, lymphatic system, the alignment of the spinal column, and the emotions. The ribs and musculature of the thorax extend over the whole area formed by the metatarsal bones on plantar and dorsal aspects of both feet.

Just as the reflex zones of the head are found in both small and larger scale on the ten toes, this rule is found to be true for the reflex zones of the neck as well. Thus the reflex zone of the neck is found on its small scale just below the pad of the large toe ventrally and fans out in its larger scale onto the ten body zones at the base joint of each toe, where it particularly includes the edge of the trapezius.

The Pelvic Girdle

The reflex zones of the pelvic girdle extend over the area of the tarsal bones and heel, up to and including the inner and outer malleoli. The region from the cuboid bone to the outer malleolus bears the reflex zones of the lateral bones and musculature of the pelvis. The area directly inferior to the inner malleolus corresponds to the symphysis pubis, while the area overlying the articulating surfaces of the fibula, talus, and tibia is the reflex zone of the hip joint.

Just as the indirect zone of the elbow could be traced from the shoulder joint, the indirect zone of the knee can be found on the fibula zone, at a point directly superior to the outer malleolus. The indirect zone of the thigh is between these two points, as well as posterior to the fibula zone.

A long-recognized reflex zone of the knee lies on the lateral rim of the heel, directly inferior to the outer malleolus. Logically, this should be a reflex zone of the pelvic region, as this area corresponds anatomically with the pelvis. However, due to the fact that this is also a reflex zone of the nerves that supply the leg, the knee can be treated here indirectly. Today's knee zones, corresponding in shape, are located on the inside and outside at the end of the thigh zones. Between them lies the kneecap.

Many years of observation have shown that in acute conditions, the reflex zone on the fibula reacts sensitively, whereas in chronic disease processes the reflex zone on the rim of the lateral heel is extremely painful as well.

REFLEX ZONES OF THE URINARY SYSTEM

In treating the reflex zones of the urinary system, the functional arrangement of the organs may be followed by proceeding from the kidney to the ureter to the bladder; or, since the bladder is not just a toneless hollow receptacle for urine but also one of the organs of excretion in that it retains and voids urine, the therapist may work from the bladder to the ureter to the kidney.

The anatomical background for the reflex zones of the kidneys lies at the base of the second and third metatarsal bones on the soles of the feet. The tendon of the hallucis longus muscle serves as an orientation line for the reflex zone of the ureter.

The tendon of the hallucis longus muscle is easily visible when the big toe is flexed dorsally; it runs from underneath the pad of the big toe

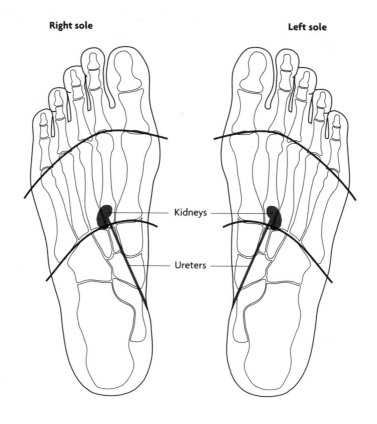

Right sole   Left sole

Kidneys

Ureters

Right inner aspect   Left inner aspect

Bladder

Sacrum with
segmental relation to bladder

Figure 9. Reflex zones of the urinary system

as far as the heel. The tendon should not be worked on while it is thus extended, but when the toes have been returned to their normal position, the tendon can be massaged along its medial corner.

The Bladder Zone

The bladder zone is represented twice. The zone immediately below the inner rim of the lateral heel is the organ zone of the bladder; the other, in the area of the lower spine, also has an effect on the bladder. Strictly speaking, this latter zone represents the nervous system of the organs of the true pelvis, and could thus also be called the corresponding zone of the bladder. The organ zone of the bladder was discovered in the early 1990s. Practice has shown that both zones often show distress and require treatment.

REFLEX ZONES OF THE ORGANS OF DIGESTION

The digestive tract begins at the mouth, whose reflex zone lies on the dorsal aspect of the big toe (see figure 10a on page 64). From here the reflex zone of the esophagus tracks proximally (on both plantar and dorsal aspects), having as its boundary the metatarso-phalangeal joint.

The stomach is best treated toward the base of the first metatarsal bone on both right and left feet. The cardia on the left foot and the pylorus on the right may be easily differentiated. The area close to the zone of the stomach opening is often marked by strong distress, which may extend to parts of the heart or diaphragm zone. In people with weak tissue who have a history of health problems, it may be useful to determine medically whether there is a case of hiatus hernia.

The three segments of the small intestine are illustrated in figure 10b (see page 65). They are not as readily distinguished in practice as in an abstract drawing; their form, length, and size alter according to their content and muscular tone. Here again a discrepancy between theoretical representation and individual feet cannot be avoided. This, however, is only of secondary importance, since it is not the name of a zone but the state of the tissue in the respective area that is of importance.

There are, however, two reliable fixed points that can be located and that serve to orient the therapist. One is the pylorus (where the stomach ends and the small intestine begins) and the other the ileocecal valve, which is the transition point from small to large intestine. Between these two points, the coils of the small intestine are found spread out over the left and right soles.

> **Note:** The zones of the small intestine are often easily recognized on visual observation of the soles when a fleshiness is noticed over the first, second, and third cuneiform bones. (See figure 2a, page 10: Bones of the feet). In West Germany, Dr. H. Mozer has frequently repositioned these bones because of some fault in their alignment.[1] We have observed a number of patients whose digestive function has markedly improved following this intervention, due to the fact that correct alignment of these bones of the feet has had a favorable influence on the reflex zones of the digestive tract.

By laying a finger across the sole of the right foot, starting from the base of the fifth metatarsal bone and directing it diagonally toward the heel, one will find (even on one's own foot), at a distance of one finger joint, the reflex zone of the appendix. Directly above this, on the dorsum of the foot, is a further reflex zone of the appendix, and this is often easier to treat. If there is greatly heightened sensitivity in this area combined with the symptoms of an acute abdomen, the patient's doctor should be informed, in case appendicitis is developing. With this zone, it is important to keep in mind that the location of the appendix can vary significantly from person to person.

The reflex zones of the pancreas are difficult to find on the feet. Since this organ cannot be easily palpated in the abdomen, neither can its reflex zone be easily differentiated from those of other organs that are related to it. Some of its functions are closely allied to those of the organs of the upper abdomen, and the pancreas is treated simultaneously with the reflex zones of the stomach, duodenum, and liver. When treating a patient with diabetes mellitus, it is necessary to work in close cooperation with the doctor, since insulin doses may sometimes need to be altered during treatment. The patient should also be instructed to take particular care to monitor sugar levels during treatment.

The reflex zones of the large intestine start on the lateral side of the right foot over the area of the tarsal bones. From here, the ascending colon tracks toward the midline of the foot, and the transverse colon lies transversely across all ten body zones of both left and right feet, as far as the lateral border of the left foot. From here the reflex zones of the descending colon track heelward, leading into the reflex zones of the sigmoid colon, rectum, and anus. This area is of particular importance, since it is often extremely painful, even when the patient does not have any known rectal pathology. It may be an indication of undiagnosed anal eczema, diarrhea, prolapsed rectum, tumor, or other pelvic disease.

Note: Experience has shown that where there is an existing disorder of the autonomic nervous system, there is an associated constriction of all the sphincters in the body, and particularly of the anal sphincter. This region (the reflex zone of the rectum and anus) should therefore be palpated in every patient where there is a suggestion of such dysfunction for verification, and if necessary, treatment.

The reflex zone of the liver is situated on the sole of the right foot and includes the reflex zone of the gallbladder at its proximal boundary on body zones 3 and 4. The reflex zone of the gallbladder is also found directly above this on the dorsum of the foot, where it is easier to locate. Note that tissue here is very sensitive to touch and can react strongly when not touched gently, including in rare cases with a hematoma.

We have observed that when a hematoma occurs on the feet following therapy, the organs that correspond to that reflex zone are overtaxed or diseased, as may also happen with the reflex zone of the gallbladder.

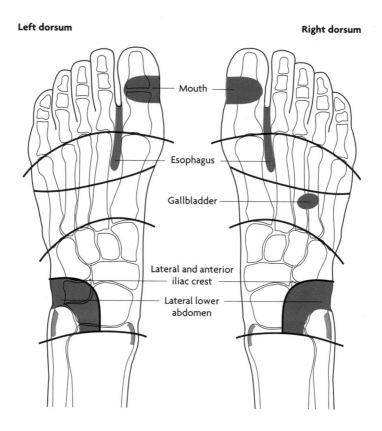

Left dorsum

Right dorsum

Mouth

Esophagus

Gallbladder

Lateral and anterior iliac crest

Lateral lower abdomen

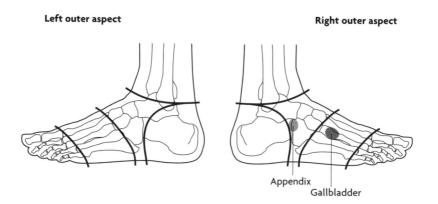

Left outer aspect

Right outer aspect

Appendix

Gallbladder

Figure 10a. Zones of the digestive organs

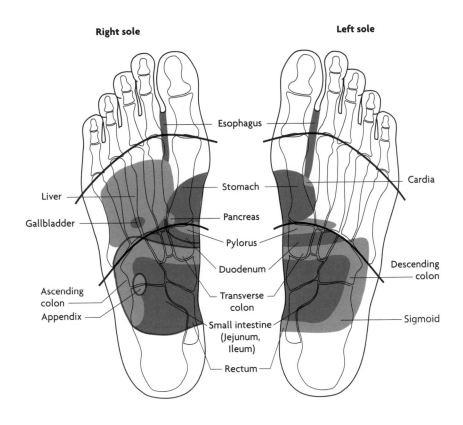

Right sole

Left sole

Esophagus

Cardia

Liver

Stomach

Gallbladder

Pancreas

Pylorus

Duodenum

Descending colon

Ascending colon

Transverse colon

Appendix

Small intestine (Jejunum, Ileum)

Sigmoid

Rectum

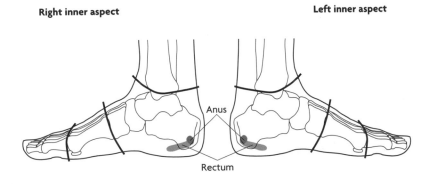

Right inner aspect

Left inner aspect

Anus

Rectum

Figure 10b. Zones of the alimentary canal

When a hematoma is present on the feet, gently include the area in your treatment in order to relieve the congestion and pain.

REFLEX ZONES OF THE ORGANS OF THE CHEST

The reflex zones of the cardiopulmonary organs are described below, and can be seen in figures 11a through 13 (pages 68–71).

Respiratory Organs

The reflex zones of the respiratory system begin, like those of the digestive tract, in the area corresponding to the nose and mouth on the dorsum of the big toe. From here the reflex zones of the trachea and bronchi are found laterally, toward the midpoint of the first and second metatarsal bones on both plantar and dorsal surfaces. From here they fan out over the large expanses that form the bronchial and lung parenchymal reflex zones, encompassing the whole area of the foot formed by the metatarsal bones.

Heart Zone

The heart has both a reflex zone of the organ and a segmental indirect reflex zone. The reflex zone of the organ is bounded on the dorsum of the foot by the area that matches the sternum and on the plantar surface of both feet by the upper part of the thoracic spine. The indirect reflex zone lies laterally on the left sole. The indirect reflex zone of the heart and the reflex zone of the shoulder girdle are identical here and also on the left dorsum, extending over the area that corresponds to the thorax, as far as the shoulder joint.

Experience has shown that it is as effective therapeutically to treat the corresponding zones of the heart as it is to treat the organ zones directly.

The rule to follow when treating the reflex zones of the heart is: "Depress hyperexcitability and stimulate flaccidity." Arndt-Schultz's basic biological precept that "weak stimuli are beneficial, strong stimuli are detrimental, very strong stimuli are harmful" has particular relevance for patients with heart disease.

When treating a patient with heart disease, the therapist should try to disassociate himself from thinking only of symptoms and consider background relationships. In many cases, the organs of digestion, the dynamic equilibrium of the spinal column, or the endocrine glands share the origin of disorder with the heart, and are therefore important for this wider and more productive way of thinking. From acupuncture we understand the dynamic effects between heart and spleen and for that reason always include the spleen when we treat the heart.

The New Solar Plexus Zone and the Diaphragm Zone

At the outset, I wish to emphasize that the previous location of the solar plexus zone is not "wrong." Strictly speaking, it is a corresponding zone, which treats the solar plexus indirectly. The area immediately below the transverse arches especially affects the upper edge of the diaphragm. Since the diaphragm has a direct relationship to respiration, work on this area has a calming effect on the vegetative nervous system.

According to Fitzgerald's ten-zone division, however, the solar plexus area is located along the midline of the body in longitudinal body zone 1, slightly in front of the lower chest and upper lumbar spine. The massage tends to be more effective when this zone is treated close to the base of the first two metatarsal bones, toward the first sphenoid bone.

As mentioned above, the "old" solar plexus zone, which lies directly beneath the transverse arches formed by the metatarsal bones in body zones 2 and 3 (see figure 10b), is very effective for treating the diaphragm. This reflex zone of the diaphragm and solar plexus provides an effective treatment for those patients who are very weak and hardly able to bear the stimulus of a traditional reflex zone massage. We have seen that such patients respond positively to repeated, gentle pressure on the "old" reflex zone of the diaphragm and solar plexus. Press gently yet firmly, to the extent that it is tolerable for the patient. This stimulation is even more effective when the pressure is applied during the patient's inhalation and released during exhalation. In this way the patient's heightened sensitivity to pain is often overcome within a few minutes.

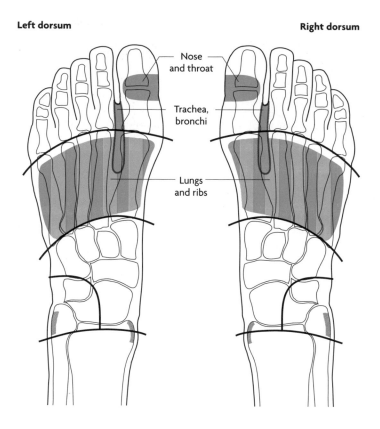

Left dorsum

Right dorsum

Nose
and throat

Trachea,
bronchi

Lungs
and ribs

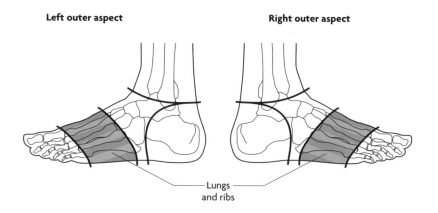

Left outer aspect

Right outer aspect

Lungs
and ribs

Figure 11a. Zones of the respiratory organs

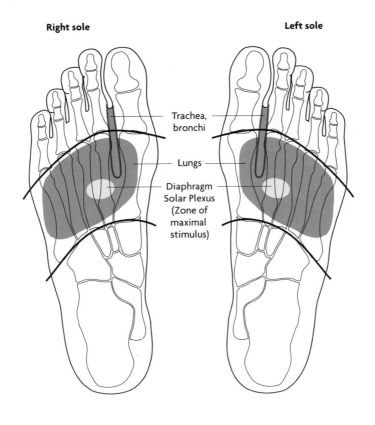

Right sole

Left sole

Trachea, bronchi

Lungs

Diaphragm
Solar Plexus
(Zone of
maximal
stimulus)

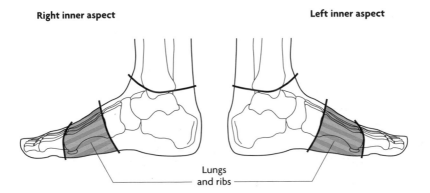

Right inner aspect

Left inner aspect

Lungs
and ribs

Figure 11b. Zones of the respiratory organs

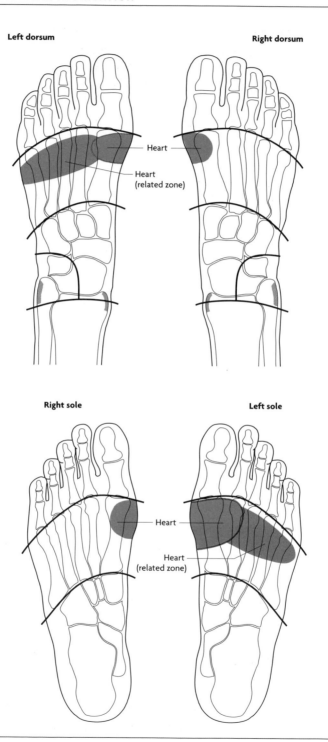

Figure 12. Zones of the heart

Right sole   **Left sole**

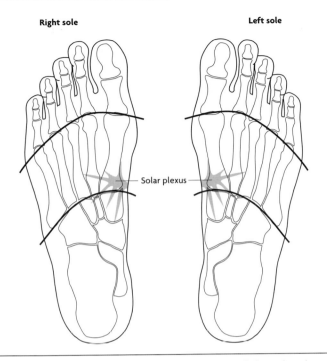

Figure 13. The new location of the reflex zone of the solar plexus

This method of general stabilization is also effectively accomplished via the "new" solar plexus zone, where a gentle touch for 20–30 seconds will usually suffice.

THE REFLEX ZONES OF THE LYMPHATIC SYSTEM

The reflex zones of the lymph vessels of the head and neck are found in the webs of the toes on both plantar and dorsal surfaces of the feet. Conspicuous among these is the reflex zone of the tonsils, situated on the lateral aspect of both big toes at their base. This zone should be treated carefully and gently, since these days it is sensitive in most people. One doesn't have far to seek for the cause of this sensitivity; the lymphatic system is the most vulnerable of the filtering systems of the human body. Personal and environmental pollution, dietary indiscretion, and the abuse of drugs and chemicals all play their part in overtaxing this system, as do

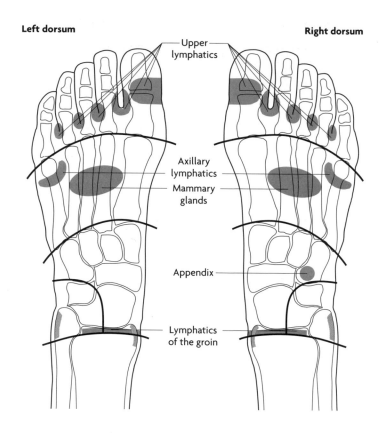

Left dorsum

Right dorsum

Upper lymphatics

Axillary lymphatics

Mammary glands

Appendix

Lymphatics of the groin

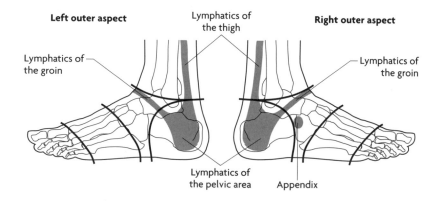

Left outer aspect

Lymphatics of the thigh

Right outer aspect

Lymphatics of the groin

Lymphatics of the groin

Lymphatics of the pelvic area

Appendix

Figure 14a. Zones of the lymphatic system

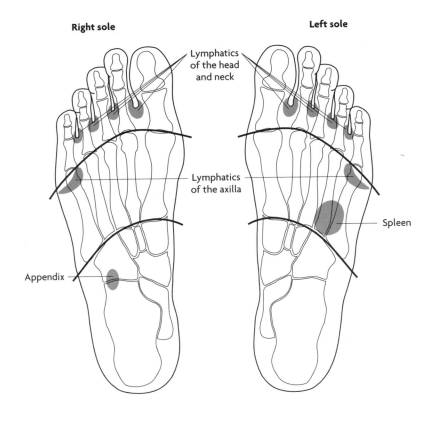

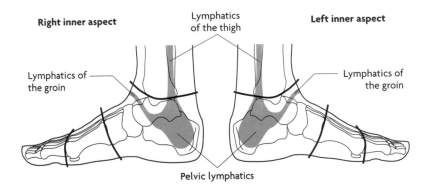

Figure 14b. Zones of the lymphatic system

illnesses that have been suppressed by unwise administration of pharmaceutical drugs.

The reflex zone of the tonsils often remains painful even when the tonsils have been surgically removed. This seems at first paradoxical, but there are two possible explanations:

1. When an organ is removed, a scar remains, and this may subsequently give rise to a painful reflex zone. (The energy field in that area is disturbed.)
2. Even after surgical removal, an organ may exert a disturbing influence on the energy field that it formerly occupied. In the same way that people who have lost a limb suffer phantom pains, all other scars and focal infections may bring about a disturbing influence on the energy fields to which they are related.

The reflex zones of the axillary lymphatics are found proximal to the shoulder joint on both plantar and dorsal surfaces. The zones for the lymphatics of the groin lie in the dorsal transverse stretch between inner and outer malleoli, between the reflex zones of the symphysis pubis and the hip joint.

The anatomical areas of the true pelvis and the upper thighs are richly endowed with lymphatic nodes and vessels, which are reflected on the medial and lateral aspects of the heel and in the area around the Achilles tendon. Lymphatic congestion of the pelvis will be accurately mirrored over this part of the heel, which must be included in the treatment of the lymphatic system.

The reflex zone of the spleen is found at the bases of the third, fourth, and fifth metatarsal bones on the plantar aspect of the left foot. According to our experience, patients who feel pain during pressure on this point might have one (or more) of the following conditions:

- Acute and chronic infections or inflammatory processes
- Blood dyscrasia, or any abnormality of blood components
- Any kind of allergy

- A predisposition to myocardial infarction (in this case the zone is often far more sensitive than would be expected)
- Stress on the upper stomach
- Emotional stress

As we can see from the list above, the reflex zone of the spleen is stressed much more frequently than is often assumed.

REFLEX ZONES OF THE ENDOCRINE SYSTEM

The reflex zones of the endocrine system are widely distributed over the feet (see figures 16a and 16b on pages 78–79), just as the endocrine system is widely distributed in the body.

The New Pituitary Zone

The zone of the pituitary gland can still be treated on the pad of the big toe, as was first suggested by Eunice Ingham in 1938. The zone is found at the center of the papilla—the concentrically arranged rings there.

Since the pad of the big toe is often pushed far to the side due to a person's weight, this spot is considered to correspond roughly to the outer lower edge of the brain but not to the anatomic location of the pituitary gland. However, practically speaking, we reach all zones of the brain—both indirectly and neutrally—from every part of the pad of the big toe, including the pituitary gland, so that its treatment on the papilla is not wrong, just imprecise.

Today, the zone can be located more precisely. Its "new" location becomes apparent when we examine our model of the ten zones according to the principle of similar shapes:

- The longitudinal zone 1, in which the pituitary gland is located, runs on each of the medial sides of the pads of the big toes. (Recall that the longitudinal zone divides into two halves at the body's rump, and can thus be found twice in the center of the feet.)
- The bone structure of the two end joints of the big toes shows

Right sole   **Left sole**

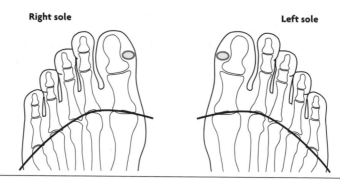

Figure 15. The new location of the pituitary gland

very clearly the shape of the so-called "Turkish saddle," in which the pituitary gland is located in the central upper part of the large brain.

Today we have relatively little practical experience with this zone of the pituitary gland, but the checks that we have been able to conduct on patients with stress or surgery in this area confirm with greater confidence its new location.

The Zone of the Thyroid

The reflex zone of the thyroid gland, which coincides in part with those of the throat and larynx, overlies the metatarso-phalangeal joints of the big toes on both the dorsal and plantar surfaces. In cases of disease, such as thyrotoxicosis, these areas should be treated with great care, since the autonomic nervous system of these patients reacts with hypersensitivity. The plantar side corresponds most closely to the area around the seventh cervical vertebra; in cases of hormonal disturbance, particularly among women, this vertebra is sometimes known as the "hormone hump," and is thus also related to the endocrine system.

The Pancreas Zone

The reflex zone of the pancreas—part endocrine gland and part organ of digestion—has already been described under the digestive tract. (See pages 61–63, 66.)

The Reflex Zone of the Adrenal Glands

In practice, it is scarcely possible to distinguish between the reflex zone of the adrenal gland and that of the kidney on either foot, since the adrenal is located so close to the superior pole of the kidney. These reflex zones are sensitive to touch, not only in cases of renal disease but also in the whole spectrum of rheumatic disease and allergies (cortisone!). This helps explain why pathological findings so often center on this zone.

Zones of the Reproductive Organs

The reflex zones of the reproductive organs are found both medially and laterally below the internal and external malleoli. On the medial aspect lie the reflex zones of the centrally located organs of the uterus and vagina, the prostate and testes. The lateral aspect contains the zones of the ovaries. As the testes descend through the inguinal canal, they may also be indirectly treated in this area.

It has been our experience that undescended testes (cryptorchidism) in young boys may be successfully treated with reflex zone therapy. It is a question of noting the background zones. (See a case history of treatment on page 146.) Some parents do not take this youthful developmental disorder seriously enough.

Care for the health and well-being of women during and after pregnancy with reflex zone therapy to the feet is particularly rewarding and beneficial to both mother and child. Normal pregnancy is not an illness; however, after much experience, no doubts remain about the benefit of such treatment.

Unfortunately, women are not always well during their pregnancies. There may be visible congestion of the veins or lymphatic vessels or problems associated with altered stance and weight-bearing, which can cause problems in the spinal column, heart, respiratory organs, or digestive tract. These conditions respond extremely well to zone therapy. It has proven best, however, to begin this therapy in the fourth month of pregnancy. Delivery and the involution of organs postpartum are usually problem-free and spontaneously accomplished, and the period of lactation may be prolonged with appropriate reflex zone massage to the feet.[2]

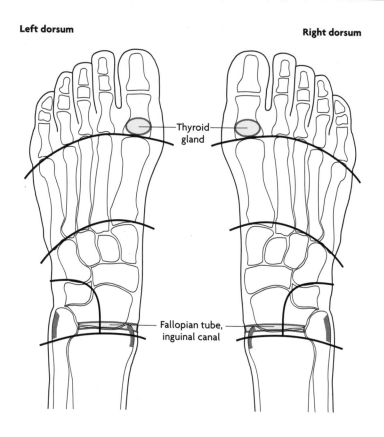

Left dorsum

Right dorsum

Thyroid gland

Fallopian tube, inguinal canal

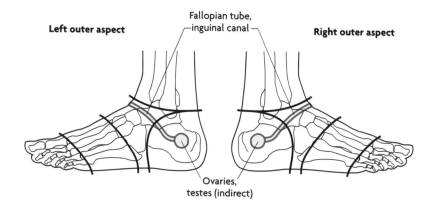

Fallopian tube, inguinal canal

Left outer aspect

Right outer aspect

Ovaries, testes (indirect)

Figure 16a. Zones of the endocrine glands

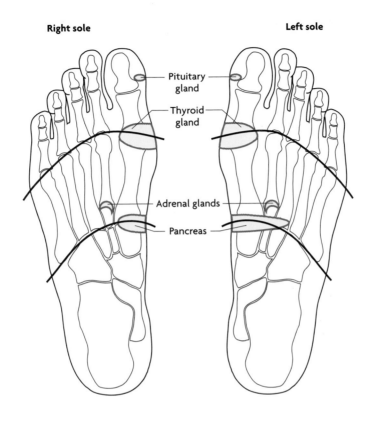

Right sole

Left sole

Pituitary gland

Thyroid gland

Adrenal glands

Pancreas

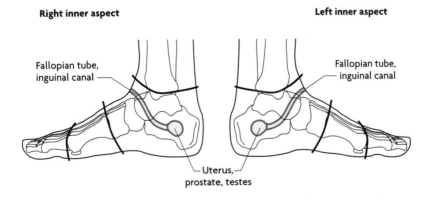

Right inner aspect

Left inner aspect

Fallopian tube, inguinal canal

Fallopian tube, inguinal canal

Uterus, prostate, testes

Figure 16b. Zones of the endocrine glands

In working with pregnant women, however, it is important to bear in mind that we never treat symptomatic zones in isolation, but always as part of a holistic therapeutic picture, paying due attention to the background that could give rise to symptoms. When the pregnancy is unstable or at risk, any decision about treatment is up to the doctor.

The reflex zones of the breasts lie centrally on the dorsum of the feet, overlying the metatarsal bones. In cases of premenstrual tension, reflex zone therapy usually relieves the symptoms until at least the next period. The known relationship between the genital area and the female breast offer the possibility of a functional treatment.

SUMMARY

When these seven groups of zones have been worked through systematically, providing the therapist with a first visual and palpable set of observations, the first assessment is concluded. It serves to guide subsequent applications of reflex zone therapy.

Since even conducting the initial assessment can cause strong reactions, it is helpful and harmonizing to carry out some balancing grips (see pages 82–83) at this point.

13

Subsequent Treatments

As noted above, only the treatments following the initial assessment mark the actual therapeutic part of reflex zone therapy. After we look briefly at the results of the initial assessment and ask the patient about reactions following the last treatment, we are able to set a new focus for each treatment. If this is not done, every treatment will see the massage of the same zones as in the initial assessment, which in all likelihood would focus excessively on the symptomatic zones. Only by taking into account any reactions between treatments (see Reactions, page 86 and also see figure 6, page 48) and then treating the zones for those reactions, can the condition of the patient be changed and improved.

The therapy is most effective when the practitioner applies pressure to the stressed zones of the foot for some seconds and then moves elsewhere, returning to these stressed zones several times during the session (usually two or three times will suffice). In this way, circulation to these zones will be improved and the tissue will normalize. This strategy also usually helps reduce any pain and hypersensitivity. Normally this can be achieved within 20–30 minutes, though there are some for whom 15 minutes will suffice and others who need 50.

The treatment grips are carried out in steps set at a distance of millimeters from one another. As soon as signs of excessive stress appear, we add balancing grips or neutral strokes. Once the condition of the reflex zones has improved markedly, the goal of the current session has been reached. The zones do not have to normalize entirely, since this process will continue until the next treatment. It is important to remember that reflex zone therapy doesn't address the symptom or the illness but primarily supports the healing and regenerative power of the patient.

One treatment series usually encompasses six, eight, or ten sessions. Many patients find it useful to continue treatment after the initial series, coming for treatments once or twice a year.

NEUTRAL STROKES AND BALANCING GRIPS

At intervals during each sequence, it is helpful to include a few breaks and gentle stroking movements. This is necessary especially when we note that we have asked too much of the patient. This can be expressed by especially intense pain on the respective zone on the foot, and/or by physical signs such as clear and sudden sweaty hands, changes in the breathing rhythm and body temperature, and so forth. (See signs of distressed zones, page 22.)

Strokes and balancing grips are also well suited to begin and end a treatment. They help create a pleasant first physical contact with the patient and help bring the course of a treatment to a quiet and calm termination.

At the end of treatment, the feet should be warm and pleasantly relaxed; a patient who returns home with cold feet cannot expect any stabilization or regeneration of his or her condition. If the feet are not comfortably warm at the end of a treatment, there are two possible reasons:

1. The dosage, intensity, and/or duration of the treatment have not been graduated according to the tolerance of the individual patient.
2. The vitality and resistance of the patient are at such a low ebb that they are inadequate to produce enough body heat to warm the patient. Therefore it may happen that, despite a thorough and

well-gauged treatment, the feet cannot be sufficiently warmed from within. In this type of case there is a place for passive warming by the judicious use of footbaths, lightboxes, hot water bottles, and so forth, but only after the treatment.

After a few treatments many patients become aware of the capacity of their own bodies to regulate and distribute body heat and at the same time realize what progress has been made up to that point.

Along with stroking and warming movements, you may occasionally introduce into the treatment a sequence of movements to relax and loosen the joints of the feet, particularly the toe joints, the metatarsal bones, and the bones of the heels.

A strong, wavelike working of the plantar parts of the base joints of the toes is a neutral stroke that is important for several reasons.

1 The articulations of the toes with the metatarsal bones correspond to the upper border of the shoulder girdle. Restoring them to normal function thus brings about a corresponding release of tension in the shoulder girdle.

2. Improving circulation in this region also has balancing and relaxing effects on other physical stresses, since this also includes the zones at the base of the toes.

3. The stability of the foot can be improved in this way, especially given the fact that for many people, the arches of the feet are crooked. A foot with a great range of motion and healthier tension, thanks to better blood circulation, helps the flexibility of the patient overall.

The middle of the foot can also be moved. Strokes around the inside and outside of the ankle (ideally with the balls of both thumbs) help to relax this often-tense tissue and can increase the range of motion of the ankle.

Stretching the heel of the foot in tune with the patient's breathing rhythm and gently touching the solar plexus zone with both thumbs also help to quickly normalize a patient who is feeling stressed by the treatment.

DIFFERENTIAL DIAGNOSIS

In patients with unclear ailments—especially around the right side of the abdomen—a differential diagnosis can be usefully complemented by a review of the zones corresponding to this area. Since only stressed, irritated zones react with pain and/or other physical signs, it is possible to clearly identify whether the patient is suffering from ailments of the right kidney, the stomach, the gallbladder, the appendix, or—in women—the right ovary. On the feet, these areas are located further apart from one another than they are on the abdomen.

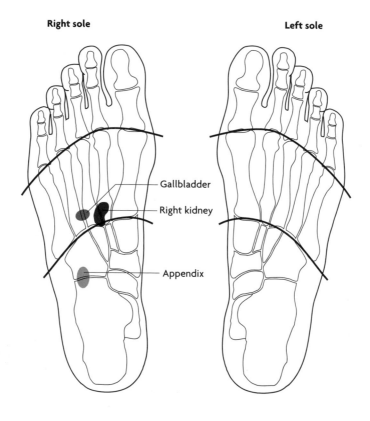

Figure 17a. Differential diagnosis of abdominal symptoms

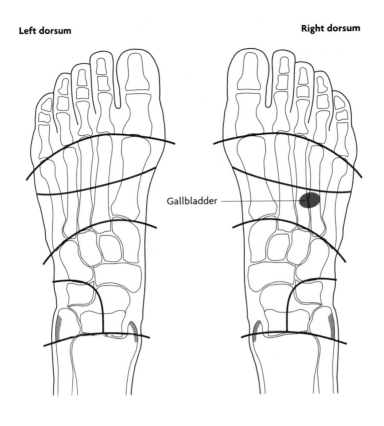

Left dorsum

Right dorsum

Gallbladder

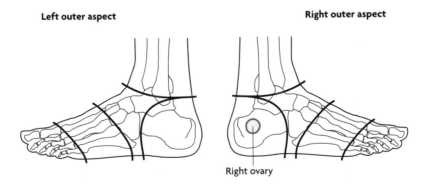

Left outer aspect

Right outer aspect

Right ovary

Figure 17b. Differential diagnosis of abdominal symptoms

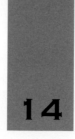

14

Reactions

Reactions during the massage enable you to observe and assess the immediate tolerance and capacity of the patient, allowing you to graduate dosage. At the commencement of therapy, the patient must be fully informed of the meaning and purpose of any reactions that may occur, either by means of a short introductory talk or a suitably prepared pamphlet, such as is used in the training school. If this step is neglected, the patient will misinterpret the reactions and may feel frightened by them.

Any change from the previous state of health—whether pleasant or disturbing, of shorter or longer duration, sharp or stimulating—is an indication of the inner healing capacity of the patient playing its part and shows that the breakdown and elimination of metabolites and toxins has begun.

The differing forms and intensities of reactions give practitioners a worthwhile lesson in observation and show the need to adapt one's massage to make it more versatile. The therapist must always bear in mind that the sick person is constantly changing—and with him, his disease picture! As practice proceeds, the therapist will need to change and modify her therapy and its practical application so that it is always in tune with each new situation. She must be able to alter with the altered needs of each patient. A standard, unchanging performance lacks vitality and becomes stale and in time ceases to be beneficial.

Note: Chronic illness cannot be directly steered toward the healing process. Instead, a regenerative detour must be sought—and guided—by the more or less evident acute phases of a patient's reactions.

REACTIONS THAT OCCUR DURING REFLEX ZONE MASSAGE

A number of reactions may accompany reflex zone massage, and they are divided into two main groups: *subjective* and *objective.*

Subjective Reactions

Subjective reactions are those that the patient feels. While a patient may or may not verbally articulate her reactions, the practitioner can often see them in the form of:

1. Changes of expression
2. Acoustic signals, including sighing, groaning, whimpering, laughing, and so forth
3. Gestures of pain, disquiet, or fear
4. Visible contraction of different muscle groups, which may affect the whole body

Objective Reactions

Objective reactions are those that would be clinically obvious to any observer, regardless of whether or not the patient is aware of them. Such reactions might include:

1. A spontanous and perhaps profuse outbreak of sweat on the palms of the hands. From this you will know that the patient will respond in a labile and hypersensitive manner to treatment.
2. Alternatively, there may be enhanced sweating of the palms in addition to outbreaks of sweat on particular areas or segments of the skin (cutaneo-visceral irritability) or over the whole body.

3. Changes in facial color, pulse rate, or saliva production.

4. A sensation of being cool or chilled, which begins at the extremities and may penetrate to the central core of the person.

5. Very occasionally a patient's inner shivering proceeds to symptoms of shock—chattering of the teeth, tetanuslike spasms, and circulatory collapse.

Both types of reaction are indicators of the personal vitality of the patient, and they demand a constant, watchful, vigilant, and alert response on the part of the therapist, whose concern must be to avoid reactions so strong that they overwhelm the resilience of the patient. This does not mean that treatment should be interrupted or concluded if any of the above-mentioned reactions occur. The reactions will, however, be factors that influence the intensity and duration of each subsequent treatment. The art of the good therapist lies in finding the right balance between his or her strength and dexterity and the capacity of the patient to benefit from this offering.

RESPONDING TO STRONG REACTIONS

If a patient responds to careful and accurately gauged treatment with unexpectedly strong reactions, the following measures will restore and balance his or her energy.

1. Remain calm and observant! A therapist who is anxious and tense will transmit her feelings of uncertainty and aggravate the condition of the patient. Remember and observe the Arndt-Schultz rule: Weak stimuli are beneficial, strong stimuli are detrimental, very strong stimuli are harmful.

2. Carry out calming strokes on both feet.

3. Take the patient's heels in the palms of your hands and pull them toward you, applying gentle tension to the legs. This will help to stimulate the breathing. Ensure that you have a cushion or support under the knees and this will enable a three-dimensional stretching of the legs and back.

4. Gently stimulate the reflex zone to the solar plexus (which is also the diaphragm) using both thumbs. (See figures 11b, page 69, and 13, page 71.)

5. Calmly hold the plantar heart zones (see figure 12, page 70) using your thumbs.

6. If necessary, apply light pressure to (and thereby regulate) the reflex zones of the following endocrine glands: the pituitary gland, which influences the activity of all the other endocrine glands; the para-thyroid glands, which share the same reflex zone as the thyroid gland and regulate blood calcium levels; and the adrenal glands, which govern the secretion of adrenalin. (See figures 16a and 16b, pages 78–79.)

The need to use point 6 above is more rare, since the patient usually recovers swiftly when his breathing and heart rate have returned to normal. Should the patient later feel cool, cold, or start shivering, apply passive warming by covering him with woolen blankets or hot water bottles. The calm, warm hands of the therapist are also effective in this warming process when placed against the soles of the feet, or used to enfold the feet, so that the patient actually feels him or herself to be "in good hands." Drinking plenty of liquids is relaxing for both parties!

In the case of such strong reactions, no further treatment should be applied. The patient should be warmly covered, undisturbed, and closely but unobtrusively observed until there is complete recovery. There is an inner, self-healing capacity present within every single person, which will work to heal the patient in combination with your treatment.

REACTIONS BETWEEN TREATMENTS

Reactions between treatments are an indication of the effects of each reflex zone massage to the feet; they are specific to each individual patient and varied in nature. They generally appear between the second and sixth treatment and usually last for a few hours, in exceptional cases for a few days. There are, of course, patients who will have one or more reactions after the first treatment, and conversely, others who will not experience them until after the fourth or sixth treatment.

Special care is needed when treating people with war injuries. Grenade and shell splinters that have become encapsulated in any organ or tissue may, as a result of reflex zone massage, move from their previous fixed position.

As long as treatment of the reflex zones is maintained at the threshold of stimulus appropriate to the patient, any reactions that occur between treatments should be regarded as desirable and anticipated signs of healing; they show the capacity of the body for self-regeneration. This holds true whether the reactions involve temporary discomfort or are accompanied by pain. They reflect an accurate picture of the patient's past and present disease picture.

When extreme reactions appear suddenly between treatments, they can be alleviated by:

- Very carefully regulating the dosage, intensity, and duration of treatment at the next visit, or
- Omitting the following treatment session to give the patient enough time and opportunity for healing regeneration

Diverse forms that reactions may take in the intervals between treatments are closely bound to the individual and the history of her disease. However, apart from this consideration, some typical reactions may occur.

- The kidneys may secrete more urine. The urine may become cloudy, with an unpleasant smell, and if left to stand for some time may develop a heavy sediment.
- Stools may increase in bulk, volume, and frequency, and also may develop an unpleasant smell. Their mucus content may be increased and they may be unusually discolored. There is frequently an increase in flatulence.
- The mucus membranes of the nasopharynx and bronchi may increase their secretions, which marks a cleansing process. The secretions may vary in color, odor, and consistency.

- There is often a marked increase in the activity of the skin, with increased perspiration that is sometimes malodorous. Occasionally a rash or pustules appear, and very occasionally a boil may erupt. Skin and tissue tonus may improve considerably, so the whole appearance is of better health and circulation.

- The patients find themselves deeply relaxed. Sleep becomes calmer and deeper. Mental and physical vitality improve. Conversely, sleep may become disturbed for a while, and dreams may be more frequent.

- Vaginal discharge may occur in women, and at times this may be so acid, concentrated, and irritating that there is inflammation and pain in the surrounding tissue.

- There may be a brief episode of fever. In general, this should be interpreted as a natural mobilization of the defenses of the body against disease and not as a sign of illness.

- Infected foci in the teeth may become painful, as may old, poorly healed scar tissue, which may also produce an exudate.

- Previous diseases that have been suppressed in the past and never truly healed may flare up for a short while. In rare instances, a whole range of past illnesses reappear for a short term before complete healing is induced.[1]

- Emotional or psychological unease may be expressed in a wide range of forms, from weeping to frank discussion of problems.

According to Paracelsus, it is Nature or the "Inner Doctor" who ordains that the organs of excretion are the main vehicle for relieving the body of stored up toxins and metabolites, some of which may have been present for many years.

It goes without saying that reactions that give rise to the suspicion of serious illness must be made known to the doctor. Responsible therapists know the boundaries and limits of their practice. It is the mark of regard for their profession that, when in doubt, they will seek medical advice once too often rather than too little. In this way, the therapist also becomes more certain of the ranges of his branch of therapy and retains the trust and confidence of his patients.

15

Using Background Zones

THE EXAMPLE OF HEADACHE PATIENTS

We can use the example of headache patients to illustrate the concept of background zones. For example, seven patients may come for therapy complaining of the same symptom, namely headache. Basic treatment for each of them would involve the reflex zones of the head, which are the symptom zones. But the next step would be to analyze what might be causing the symptom in each patient and treat the zones corresponding to those causes.

With headaches, the following background zones must be considered:

- The alimentary tract
- Altered dynamics of the spinal column, particularly in the cervical vertebrae
- Teeth and sinuses
- The genitourinary tract
- The solar plexus and diaphragm, whose reflex zones may be a factor in conditions of stress and psychic disturbance
- The organs of respiration

In reality, however, it is rare to find only one of these background zones playing a role. More frequently, we see combinations of causes, each of which should be treated. Since every patient will undergo an initial assessment that will test all zones for stress, it is possible that additional zones besides the ones listed above will be found to be in need of treatment.

To illustrate this phenomenon more clearly, the following pages show six examples of headache, each with different background zones. See figures 18a–23b (pages 94–105).

SUMMARY

The illustrations of these six headache patients show that reflex zone treatment can lead beyond the foot, away from isolated thinking focused on symptoms and pathological labels, and toward a more holistic view of a patient. This includes paying due attention to his or her psychological and emotional state.

There is a dynamic relationship between body and emotions, such that imbalances in one can affect the other, and vice versa. For example,

- A painful reflex zone of the gallbladder gives not only the impression of a physical state of illness, which may be confirmed in the laboratory but also that in such a person the gall "overflows."
- A painful reflex zone of the shoulder girdle gives, on the surface, evidence of tension in this area, but behind this there is frequently an additional psychic stress, so that the patient "carries a heavy burden on his shoulders."
- Another patient has an extremely sensitive zone of the intestine, suffers from flatulence, and has little appetite despite careful selection of diet—all of which indicate an organic problem. Such symptoms frequently disappear spontaneously when the patient is better able to "digest" the difficulties in his life.

Note: While the knowledge of the relationship between body and psyche is widely known, it has to be realized anew by each and every person and in every treatment to keep it alive. Whether, when, and in what way the therapist can discuss these relationships with a patient depends on the therapist's experience and sensitivity.

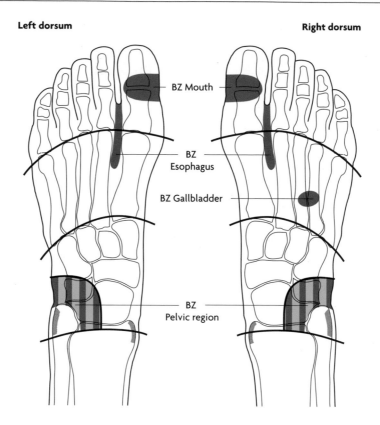

Left dorsum

Right dorsum

BZ Mouth

BZ
Esophagus

BZ Gallbladder

BZ
Pelvic region

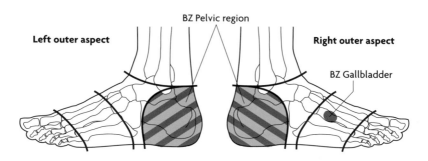

BZ Pelvic region

Left outer aspect

Right outer aspect

BZ Gallbladder

Background Cause: Digestive tract disorder

Symptoms occur in: Zones of the head

Background Zones (BZ): Stomach, cardiac sphincter, and pyloric sphincter; the three segments of the small intestine; large intestine, particularly the ileocecal valve; (transition from small to large intestine), sigmoid, rectal, and anal areas; pancreas; liver and gallbladder; pelvic regions (which share a reflex relationship with organs in the lower abdomen).

Figure 18a. Patient with headache, example 1

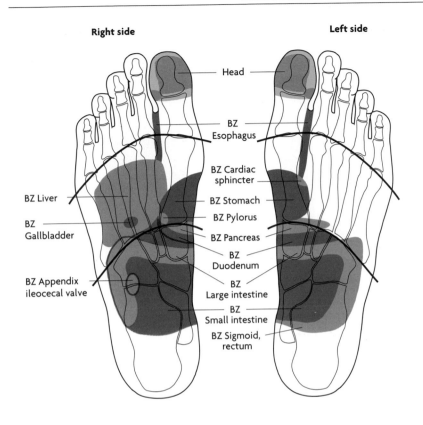

Right side

Left side

Head

BZ
Esophagus

BZ Cardiac
sphincter

BZ Liver

BZ Stomach

BZ
Gallbladder

BZ Pylorus

BZ Pancreas

BZ
Duodenum

BZ Appendix
ileocecal valve

BZ
Large intestine

BZ
Small intestine

BZ Sigmoid,
rectum

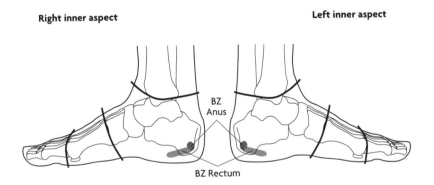

Right inner aspect

Left inner aspect

BZ
Anus

BZ Rectum

Figure 18b. Patient with headache, example 1

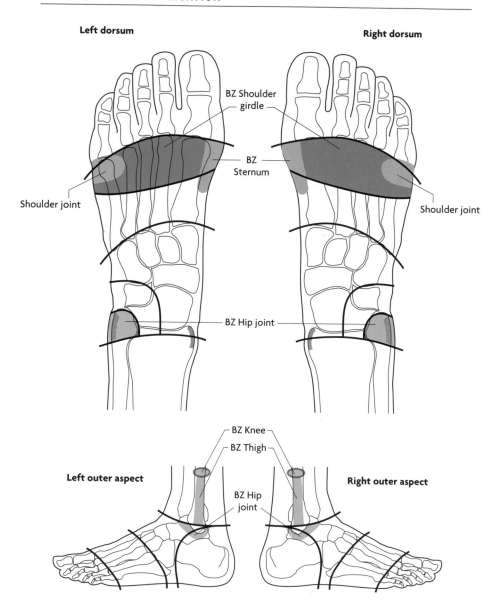

Background Cause: Disturbed dynamic equilibrium of the vetebral column

Symptoms occur in: Zones of the Head

Background Zones (BZ): Neck; entire vertebral column, particularly that area where the disorder is most pronounced (usually cervical vertebrae); shoulder girdle and shoulder joints; hip joints and knee joints.

Figure 19a. Patient with headache, example 2

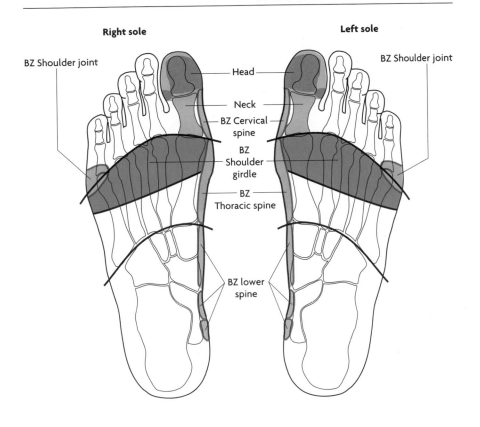

Right sole

Left sole

BZ Shoulder joint

BZ Shoulder joint

Head

Neck

BZ Cervical spine

BZ Shoulder girdle

BZ Thoracic spine

BZ lower spine

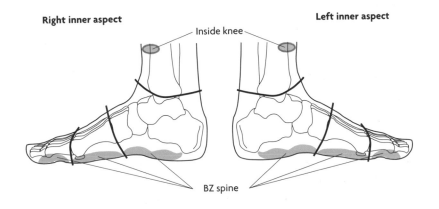

Right inner aspect

Left inner aspect

Inside knee

BZ spine

Figure 19b. Patient with headache, example 2

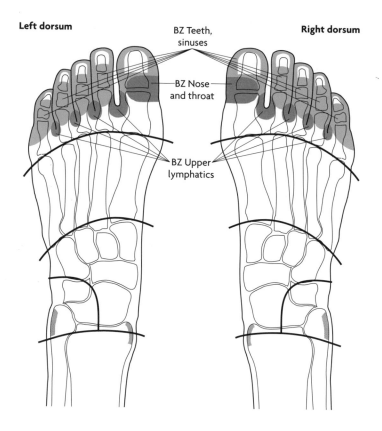

Left dorsum

BZ Teeth,
sinuses

BZ Nose
and throat

BZ Upper
lymphatics

Right dorsum

Background Cause: Disorder of jaw and teeth

Symptoms occur in: Zones of the Head

Background Zones (BZ): Sinuses, teeth; nose and throat; lymphatic channels of the head and neck; spleen (as in all infections); appendix

Figure 20a. Patient with headache, example 3

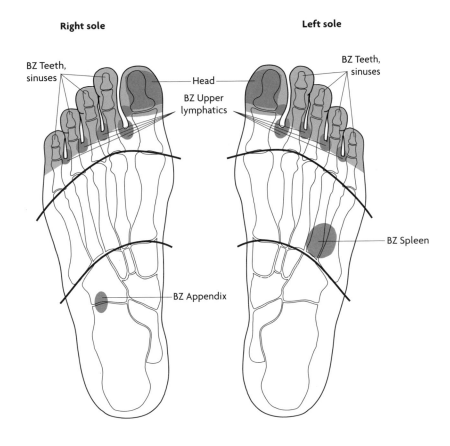

Right sole

Left sole

BZ Teeth, sinuses

BZ Teeth, sinuses

Head

BZ Upper lymphatics

BZ Spleen

BZ Appendix

Figure 20b. Patient with headache, example 3

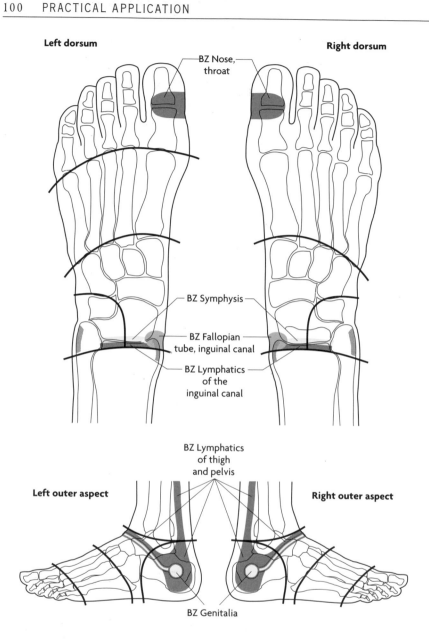

Left dorsum

Right dorsum

BZ Nose, throat

BZ Symphysis

BZ Fallopian tube, inguinal canal

BZ Lymphatics of the inguinal canal

BZ Lymphatics of thigh and pelvis

Left outer aspect

Right outer aspect

BZ Genitalia

Background Cause: Disease of urogenital tract

Symptoms occur in: Zones of the Head

Background Zones (BZ): Kidneys, ureters and bladder; genitalia; lymphatic pathways in the groin and in the head and neck; lower spine; pelvis and symphysis, spleen

Figure 21a. Patient with headache, example 4

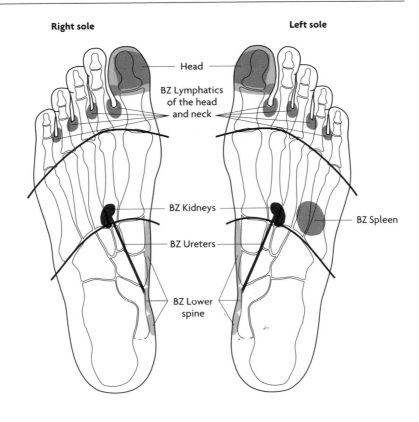

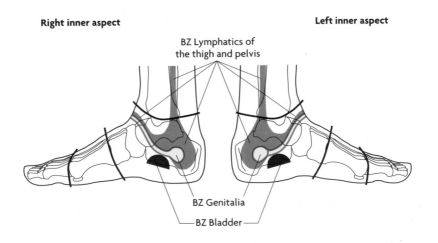

Figure 21b. Patient with headache, example 4

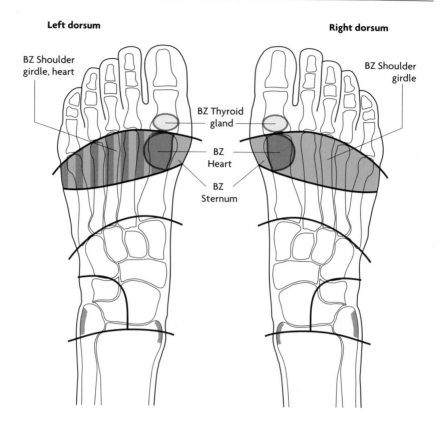

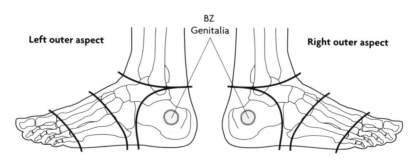

Background Cause: Disorder of autonomic nervous system, possibly of the psyche; stress

Symptoms occur in: Zones of the head

Background Zones (BZ): Solar plexus (the same zone as the diaphragm); all endocrine glands: pituitary, thyroid, adrenal glands, genitalia; shoulder girdle, neck (because of the "burden the sick person has to carry on their shoulders"); heart, sternum, spleen.

Figure 22a. Patient with headache, example 5

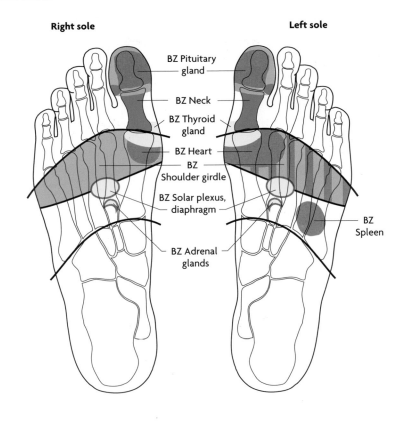

Right sole

Left sole

BZ Pituitary
gland

BZ Neck

BZ Thyroid
gland

BZ Heart

BZ
Shoulder girdle

BZ Solar plexus,
diaphragm

BZ
Spleen

BZ Adrenal
glands

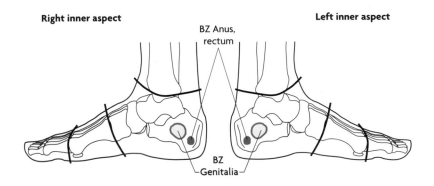

Right inner aspect

Left inner aspect

BZ Anus,
rectum

BZ
Genitalia

Figure 22b. Patient with headache, example 5

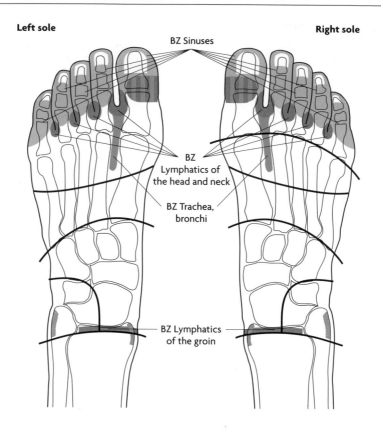

Left sole

BZ Sinuses

Right sole

BZ Lymphatics of the head and neck

BZ Trachea, bronchi

BZ Lymphatics of the groin

Left outer aspect

Right outer aspect

BZ Genitalia

Background Cause: Respiratory tract infection

Symptoms occur in: Zones of the head

Background Zones (BZ): Nose and throat; lymphatics of the head and neck; bronchi; lungs; sinuses; spleen (as in all infections); pelvic organs (bladder, genitalia) because of their reflex relationships to the nose and throat; liver and kidneys (to aid elimination of metabolites).

Figure 23a. Patient with headache, example 6

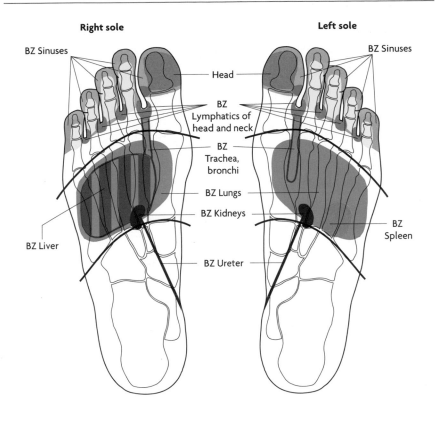

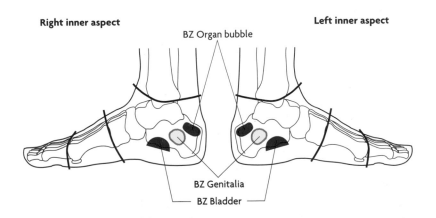

Figure 23b. Patient with headache, example 6

The question of the effectiveness of reflex zone therapy of the feet always also includes the question of the reaction of the patient. Depending on the patient's own readiness for internal and external order, abilities and possibilities grow. It can be said that many diseases can be treated but not all people can, since some lack the necessary will to be restored to health and well-being.

As a differentiated manual form of treatment, reflex zone therapy of the foot meets a healthy natural need on the part of both therapists and patients. Patients are, in many cases, already seeking healing from unorthodox forms of medicine and are not wholly dependent on the apparatus of modern medicine. They will come to appreciate the fact that a balanced form of therapy stimulates their entire energy field—including the psyche—with beneficial effects.

The task of an aspiring practitioner extends far beyond learning and applying the actual "technique" of the grip sequence. With skilled, imaginative, and informed reflex zone massage, the whole person can be treated. The therapist acquires a broad view of medicine and learns to apply his skills with compassion on multiple levels:

- On the rational level by learning new theoretical foundations and relationships
- On the emotional level by developing healthy empathy toward patients and their ailments (This is different from personal empathy, which lacks the necessary professional distance but includes attentive care.)
- On the physical level through the balanced use of strength

Thus the therapist helps patients on one part of the journey from illness to health and can encourage them to take responsibility for their health. The therapist will exercise his profession with greater commitment and devotion when he is engaged in a sensibly planned total regime and is not just treating isolated parts of the patient at random.

16

Interpreting Stressed Reflex Zones

Healthy tissue possesses good tonus and feels well circulated. In a healthy reflex zone with good circulation, the probing hand of the therapist invokes an impulse in the nerve endings of the feet that is no different from that of a similar tissue displacement in any other healthy part of the body. It should not be painful.

When the reflex zone is abnormal, however, the patient reacts to the impulse of pressure, no matter how carefully graduated, simply because it causes pain. The occurrence of pain and indications from the autonomic nervous system during reflex zone work on the foot are reliable guides to treatment. The nonpainful signs of the autonomic nervous system that indicate an irritation of the reflex zones are described more extensively in chapter 5.

There are distinct grades to the quality of pain a patient may feel:

1. The most surprising sensation is that of a sharp, pricking pain, usually concentrated in an area the size of a pinhead, and often so intense that the patient wonders if it was made by a sharp object or a fingernail. This pain is usually experienced in the toes and heels.
2. Another kind of pain is experienced in the tissues. It is frequently felt over a broad area, and it is not uncommon to hear this pain

described as a "pain that is accompanied by a sense of well-being."

3. Exceedingly sharp pain is experienced in the webs of the toes or on the lateral aspect of the fifth metatarsal bones, usually in association with the milking or wringing movements used here.

We make sure not to see the pain of our patients as an enemy that we are fighting. To this end, dose the therapeutic grips in gradations that allow your patients to deal with the pain. They will experience an improvement in their ailments as soon as they overcome their pain.

At the same time, do not confuse the patient's subjective accounts with your own objective findings resulting from visual and physical examination. Your findings will differ from his because:

- The patient describes only symptoms and often thinks this is the illness.

- He sometimes forgets the essentials and emphasizes the less essential.

- He mentions none of his latent problems, since he is as yet unaware of them.

- Because of severe afflictions in a particular organ or system, pain in other places that is less acute, or symptoms that are less troublesome, are often glossed over. These first come to light when the initial strong pain has diminished. At the point in the treatment sequence when patients become aware of pain that had previously been ignored, they come to believe that the therapy made them "sicker" than they were before.

Most patients believe that their illness commenced with the first appearance of the initial symptoms. "Yesterday evening I caught a cold," or "On Sunday the rheumatism in my shoulder started playing up." However, this is not the truth of the matter. Every illness is preceded by a prodromal or incubation period, which may last for days, weeks, months, or years. Only when the patient cannot successfully maintain homeostasis from within do the acute and later the chronic phases of the illness become apparent. It is only in accidents that injury and signs and symptoms occur simultaneously, and even here it is worth thinking about whether the accident had not already been in the making on "other" levels.

The beginner will find it difficult at times not to attach more importance to what the patient says than to what she has discovered as a result of her own examination. From the very first reflex zone massage of the feet, therapists must practice self-reliance, and will in due course come to see the subjective statements made by their patients as only one part of their clinical findings.

A patient may complain of a stomach disorder, for example, and believe that she is otherwise "quite healthy." Objective palpation of the feet, however, reveals that in addition to the stomach, the small intestine, the liver, the cervical spine, the solar plexus, and the right knee respond abnormally in their reflex zones. If the therapist is uncertain of her ground, she will not know which finding is correct.

Note: In every case, visual and palpable observations arising from examination are more valid than any mention of symptoms, since we are not treating an isolated illness, but the sick person in her entirety, in all her aspects.

17

Duration of Treatment

The number of reflex zone massages that will be necessary for each individual patient cannot be determined or stated with exactitude at the commencement of treatment. The patient's background and the immediate general condition of the whole organism are too complex to allow this. In addition, there are many internal and external influences that can affect a patient during the course of treatment.

Any of the following factors may lengthen the duration of treatment:

- Climatic stimuli, including gale-force winds or the commencement of cold wet weather, for example
- Changes in diet, including temporary indulgences adopted during travel or office events, or eating highly spiced and seasoned foods experimentally or occasionally
- Alterations in the wake-sleep rhythm, whether they're occasioned by night duty, shift work, anxiety, or overexcitement
- Continual changes in the patient's personal biorhythms from the active to the passive phase and vice versa
- Latent illness, a quiescent phase, or the incubation period of an infectious disease
- Psychic or emotional trauma in the family or at work

- Geopathic stress: from geographic areas that exert a strong influence, or from the mechanization of the environment in one's place of work or at home. Consider the prevalence of radios, digital alarm clocks and watches, television, too many mirrors, and plastic or synthetic fabrics.
- Poisons in the air, in the water, in cleaning products, in food, in synthetic fabrics, and even impregnated in dusters and cleaning cloths

DECIDING ON A COURSE OF TREATMENT

As long as positive reactions result from your treatment, there is value in continuing that treatment. This holds true even when ten to twelve treatments have been completed.

The total number of treatments needed depends most importantly on the ability of the patient's body to react to treatment, as well as on his overall vitality and capacity for adjusting to changes. It's also important to consider the background that gave rise to the illness, the patient's biological age, and the manner in which the patient conducts his or her life.

Sometimes a single reflex zone massage to the feet restores essential order to a dysfunction of some years' standing. This does not mean that the treatment should be discontinued, as a short series of foot treatments will have the effect of stabilizing and consolidating that person's condition.

When no particular disorder is apparent, a short course of treatment can be repeated after an interval of a year or so or whenever the patient feels it to be necessary.

18

Treatment Combinations

When reflex zone therapy does not fully produce the desired improvement in the patient's condition, it may be necessary to add another form of treatment as well. As a natural therapy, reflex zone massage combines well with other natural healing disciplines.

Combinations that have proven especially effective in practice are:

- All naturopathic health practices that encourage detoxification of the body fluids—especially the blood and lymph. These include the regime of fasting for health and in order to improve intestinal function, as advocated by Dr. F. X. Mayr;[1] mild abstinence,[2] and fasting according to the rules laid sown by Schroth and Felke and by Buchinger.
- Hydrotherapy as advocated by Kneipp,[3] Kuhnet,[4] Priessnitz, and Schlenz.
- Similar proven manual therapies, such as acumassage, connective tissue massage, chiropractic and chirogymnastics, classical massage, manual lymph drainage, and shiatsu.
- Herbal and homoeopathic remedies, acupuncture.
- Dietary measures such as those advocated by Hay,[5] F. X. Mayr, and Waerland.

- Deep breathing exercises, gymnastics, postural correction according to Alexander, Feldenkrais, Glaser, Middendorf, Qi Gong, Schaarschuch/Haase,[6] Schlaffhorst-Andersen, and Schroth (for treatment of scoliosis).

- Treatment of a disordered energy field, including: (a) treatment of scars through neural therapy; (b) treatment of infected foci in teeth and sinuses using proven biochemical methods without recourse to chemical treatments; and (c) eliminating "geopathic" irritations and stimuli from the places where one works and lives. An excess of cement, steel, glass, and artificial fibers creates an atmosphere that is antithetical to healthy living.

Reflex zone therapy of the feet may also act beneficially on a disturbed field other than the feet, such as the teeth and body scars. Patients often mention that during or after a reflex zone massage, they feel a prickling, pulling, or light stabbing sensation in a scar. In rare cases, massage to an area of the feet that corresponds to a scarred part of the body brings about a spontaneous hematoma over or around the actual scar tissue. As the hematoma reabsorbs, any pain or contraction of the scar diminishes.

Reflex zone therapy has proven effective for speeding healing after a tooth extraction or dental surgery, for periodontitis, and as general complement to a holistic approach to dental care. Of course, it is important to pay attention to a healthy diet, since this plays a major role in the maintenance of healthy teeth.

When a combination of treatments is being carried out, they must be coordinated with one another. It is dangerous for therapeutic stimuli to follow one another too quickly, and the effect of one may cancel out the effect of another.

If a warm footbath has been taken immediately before reflex zone massage, the observations you make visually and as a result of palpation will be distorted due to recent thorough warming, particularly if chemical bath salts were added to the water. If passive warming of the feet is necessary, it is best done at the end of treatment.

Note for Beginners: It is less effective, and even harmful, to apply the different grips indiscriminately to unselected areas of the feet. Use firm discipline in confining, restricting, and limiting yourself to that which is effective. Anyone wishing to employ more than one manual therapy discipline in a single treatment must indeed know what he or she is doing!

19

Feet and Hands

A legitimate question is frequently asked: Why do most therapists—including Dr. Fitzgerald and Eunice Ingham—concern themselves more with the feet than with the hands? According to the ten-zone division of the body, it should in theory be possible to perform the same therapy on the hands. Besides which, the hands are better cared for than the feet, they are more accessible for treatment, and, as can be seen from their anatomical structure, they are softer and more flexible.

Despite these apparent advantages, practice in fact dictates unequivocally that treatment is more effective on the feet. The feet have a reciprocal connection with the earth, and they may be imagined as two poles, responsible for the equalization of mankind's electromagnetic field. The feet have often been likened to the roots of a plant, which we know have a great capacity for regeneration.

Because they are generally so neglected and ill cared for, the feet respond gratefully to care and treatment, although they are still the orphans of health care. When comparing the hands with the feet, we assign to the hands greater importance in relation to the thinking and feeling areas of life. Hands make music, write, caress, pray, model, and gesticulate: so that even on a physical level they fulfill a different function than the feet. The feet, on the other hand, give us the feeling of being "grounded." It is from the substantial base of the surface of the earth that we learn to raise ourselves and walk erectly.

In susceptible people, cold feet have long been incriminated as a predisposing factor in illnesses such as tonsillitis, laryngitis, bronchitis, cystitis, pyelitis, and otitis, as well as other acute and chronic ailments. For this reason, it is all the more important to have a range of therapies and practices for improving the health of the feet—and thereby of the person as a whole.

The healthy stimulus of walking barefoot on the beach or on grass is generally held to be strengthening and beneficial to the circulation of the feet. There is also a growing interest in shoes that do not cramp and confine the feet, such as Kneipp, Berkeman, and Birkenstock sandals in Europe, and Nature shoes in England.

It was not without reason that Sebastian Kneipp stressed the value of treatment of the feet. Walking on dewy grass, treading in water, and wearing vinegar-soaked stockings were among the treatments he advocated; it is unfortunate that these valuable treatment measures have been neglected.

There are many other effective treatments for feet. In our experience, the Schiele footbath (a temperature-raising bath), the Schluter footbaths, and, more recently, the remarkably curative results achieved by the French herbalist Maurice Mességué [1] are all extremely beneficial.

In summary, practice has proven that while treatment of the reflex zones of the hands is complementary to treatment of the reflex zones of the feet, emphasis should remain on treatment of the feet. These neglected surfaces may reveal surprising insights into the open secret of the enduring laws of nature and biological renewal.

20

The "Right" Age
for Reflex Zone Massage

Over and over again, we hear that those over the age of seventy and under the age of three or four years are advised against having this treatment. The argument given is that they will not easily be able to bear the pain of reflex zone therapy. What is overlooked is that it is not the treatment that "gives" them pain. Pain is not an abstract quality. It has already assumed a personal quality by being present in a sick person.

As far as the therapy is concerned, the individual pain threshold is readily discerned through the reactions that manifest during treatment. Every sick person, regardless of age, suffers from that pain that directly relates to his illness and must be physically and emotionally endured. Adjusting the dosage of treatment on painful areas of the foot is a basic requirement that all therapists should heed when working with patients.

Years of practical experience have shown that elderly people are especially responsive to this form of therapy and will respond amazingly quickly and positively to natural healing stimuli. Often their regenerative ability is as good as, if not better than, that of younger people, who have had greater exposure to environmental and nutritional pollution.

As most people in the West enjoy a materially higher standard of living today than in previous decades, it is even more imperative that they should be well cared for in their old age, so that they may pass the remainder of their life span relatively free of affliction and able to depend on their own strength. Even when no acute infirmity is evident, one or two courses of reflex zone massage each year is an appropriate prophylactic measure for both the young and the elderly.

As far as the treatment of children is concerned, while it is true that—depending on their age—young children cannot verbally describe their pain, they do have very clear ways of showing the limits of their tolerance, with facial and acoustic signals. The autonomic nervous system also reports if the therapeutic stimulus was too strong, for example through moist hands or a change in breathing. Finally, children learn to deal with painful or unpleasant stimuli from the day they are born, and often even in the womb. Thus, a reflex zone massage to the feet may be given in the first few days of life. Infants and children are grateful patients. Most of them have a more uncomplicated understanding of healing than adults and are far less demanding than their overindulged elders realize.

Over the years, many interesting observations have been made regarding children. Even those who are relatively healthy and free of ailments often manifest abnormal zones on their feet where we least expect to find them. The explanation for these is often found only after a visual and palpatory examination of the parents. Painful zones on the feet of parents and their offspring display an amazing inherited disposition to illness. The inference is that such inherited predispositions are already evident in childhood, and may be amenable to treatment by massage of the reflex zones of the feet at that time.

A prominent finding in children is increased sensitivity in the lymphatic reflex zones. This is presumably in part due to faulty diet. Some mothers find it troublesome to breastfeed, and in some cases may dismiss it as being old-fashioned. Later on, products made up of white refined flour and sugar form too great a proportion of the child's daily nutrition. In addition, the repeated administration of proprietary medicines instead of healing remedies and of too many immunizations also plays a part in weakening a child's system. For children with resistance that has been thus weakened, reflex zone massage is effective in stimulating and building them up.

21

Emollients and Foot Aids

There are a multitude of foot products available that people imagine will enhance their reflex zone therapy treatments. In fact, treatment tends to do better unadorned, though some of the products do have other benefits.

EMOLLIENTS

No emollient should be used during reflex zone massage to the feet. However, the therapist may apply an herbal ointment, oil, or essential oil to stimulate the circulation at the end of treatment.

Beware of chemical footsprays! They clog the pores and prevent the feet from ridding themselves (and the rest of the body) of excretions from the sweat glands. Suppressing the ability of the body to sweat through the feet is unwise. Excessive sweating, particularly if malodorous, is an indication of imbalance that should be heeded. In fact, the therapist may gather much valuable information from patients who present with different, strange odors given off by the feet. If the smells are markedly offensive during treatment, a pure cologne water may be applied. The patient should be informed that shoes, socks, and stockings of synthetic materials increase the likelihood of sweating, and the likelihood of offensive odors because they don't allow for local ventilation. Patients with persistent unpleasant foot odor should be advised to change socks and stockings daily, and to take daily footbaths, to which sea salt or cider vinegar may be added.

MECHANICAL AIDS FOR THE FEET

It is now possible to purchase a variety of "foot aids," such as rollers, mats, spheres, brushes, platters made of various materials, and gadgets that are operated partially or wholly by electricity. While such tools are often attractive, it is important for patients to know exactly what their potentials and limits are.

The use of such implements is neither harmful nor unprofitable, but they are sometimes ascribed with a potential that they simply cannot have. It is like comparing the inadvertent prick of a finger by a sewing needle with the practice of acupuncture, or a wetting of the feet with hydrotherapy—so faintly do such implements resemble specific treatment. At best they tap the symptoms of the patient.

Such aids are therefore only useful when they are recognized for what they are. They can promote circulation and lymphatic drainage in the feet. They may warm you up, and they may strengthen and relax weakened or taut muscles in the feet, making them more elastic—but only when they are rightly employed and not when they are overused.

In short, these tools are not to be mistaken for instruments of reflex zone therapy. That is the realm of the responsible therapist who knows why, where, when, how strongly, and for how long to work on the feet.

Imagine, for example, a person with a heart or kidney disorder, whose organ disease has resulted in a marked sensitivity in the corresponding reflex zones of the feet. Using one of the above-mentioned implements could do more harm than good for such a patient. The patient or practitioner may not be aware of the first principle of this work—sedate hyperactivity and stimulate flaccidity. Or they may find themselves concerned solely with symptoms rather than broadening their horizon to consider causes.

When learning a foreign language, nobody would think that reading individual words in a foreign script amounts to mastery of the language; we know that the relationship of the words to one another is what gives them meaning. The same applies to these foreign "languages" of therapy.

22

Self-Treatment

Anyone who is mobile, whose joints are flexible, and who can easily raise their legs to the level of the trunk can treat the reflex zones of their own feet. There are certain points to remember during self-treatment, particularly when the person has not been trained in this discipline.

- Self-treatment is not more than general health care or a form of first-aid (in the same way that one might use Kneipp hydrotherapy at home).
- Because one is both patient and therapist at the same time, the benefit of influence exerted by the personality of the therapist is absent.
- Relaxation is difficult to achieve, since, of necessity, one must raise one's feet.
- The characteristic indications of adequate treatment—like sweating, coolness, inner warmth—cannot be assessed objectively. Sweating may be the result of the exertion of self-treatment rather than from having correctly measured the dosage. It is also difficult to observe the cooling of one's own extremities.
- Hands that are unpracticed soon tire. Implements such as wooden pestles, rubber mats, or vibrators give no clue to the differing states of tissue in the feet.

- Anyone who is inexperienced or inexpert in observing the progress of disease is unable to assess the reaction phase correctly. They are inclined to lay undue emphasis on looked-for reactions and to minimize (through ignorance) the actual state of the disease, which is truly the province of the doctor. They are usually swayed by the obvious symptoms because they do not understand the interaction of all systems.

- The initial enthusiasm that people feel when they first come into contact with this interesting method often falls off into one of two extremes—either a resignation and outright condemnation when it does not always and immediately offer relief, or fanaticism, which breeds the little "wonder doctor" who instantly markets a diagnosis and gives advice that is presented as a total and instant cure.

Notwithstanding the above somewhat limiting points, good self-treatment can be helpful in situations where trained therapists are not available. In such cases, the ideal working team would consist of:

- A well-informed and interested doctor, who will oversee the patient's treatment.

- A responsible practitioner of reflex zone therapy to supervise the patient's self-treatment. This practitioner should be educated in practice and theory and should have insight into the constantly changing circumstances of the patient's life.

- A competent, conscientious podiatrist.

- A patient who is prepared to cooperate and who is open-minded and willing to give the benefit of the doubt to a treatment of which he knows nothing.

PART THREE

CASE HISTORIES

23

Treatment of Specific Ailments

CASE HISTORIES

This section of the book has been put together from written and verbal accounts of therapists and participants at the seminars I have taught. Students have continued to share with me reports from their own practice, some of which I share here, along with some stories of my own.

Important! The experiences and progress during treatment described on the pages that follow will never be exactly reproduced in another person with similar symptoms. Each person will react individually and differently.

One of the basic principles of reflex zone massage to the feet is reiterated here: It is not the illness that we treat, but the entire sick person.

ABDOMINAL CRAMPS

A housewife, aged thirty-three, had suffered for a long time from abdominal cramps, which she found unbearable. Besides the painful reflex zones of the entire digestive tract, which were reactive on palpation, she had a wart 0.5 cm thick on the sole of her right foot, over the area of the small intestine.

This woman experienced some relief of her symptoms after the second reflex zone massage. The wart became visibly smaller with each successive treatment and the cramps were less painful. By the time she had had seven massages, her bowel movements had returned to normal, she had less flatulence, and the pain had completely ceased. After twelve treatments, circulation in the area where the wart had formed was normal, and a year later she reported that she continued to feel well.

ACUTE EARACHE

When two-year-old Michael was brought by his mother for treatment, he was crying and in obvious pain, rubbing his right ear with his fist. The ear was red and inflamed, but a closer inspection was not possible since he was in too much pain.

A firm hold was maintained on the reflex zone to the right ear for two minutes (using the sedation grip), and the child went to sleep in his mother's arms. He has had no recurrence of his earache. The first treatment was followed by a series of twelve weekly treatments to consolidate the result. In these treatments, the kidney and intestinal zones were found to be distressed.

ALLERGY

A shop assistant, thirty-five years old, suffered from repeated allergic rashes, which were at times accompanied by impaired consciousness. With each attack, she had to spend several days in the hospital. By chance, a therapist who had had a similar experience and had been trained in reflex zone therapy was present on one of these occasions and examined her feet.

The reflex zones for the lymph glands, the endocrine glands, the liver, and the spleen were extremely sensitive. Fifteen minutes after the initial examination and treatment, the rash, itching, and lapses in consciousness became less marked, and the patient fell into a deep and refreshing sleep. A further eight treatments followed at intervals of three to four days, after which the reflex zones were relatively painless, and the allergy did not reappear.

ARTHROSIS

A carpenter, fifty-two years old, came into the clinic three years ago with severe pain and limited range of motion in his left knee. He received foot wraps and in the following weeks reflex zone therapy of the feet.

The zones of the urinary tract, the stomach, the lower spine, and the left and right knees were painful. Within fifteen treatments, the symptoms decreased noticeably in severity. Today the patient is back to his daily run, without being bothered by his knee.

ATAXIA

A six-year-old child with Rhesus negative blood suffered from ataxia and almost unintelligible pronunciation due to excessive salivation. It had been stated that she would have to enter a special school, although she was not mentally handicapped.

On palpation, all the reflex zones of the head were taut and tense, and those of the thyroid gland, urogenital tract, and the lymph glands of the throat and pelvis were very sensitive to touch. After the second treatment, the child's hands were noticeably more still, salivation started to diminish, and her speech and ataxia started to improve.

She had fifteen treatments in two months and subsequently passed the entrance test to the local elementary school. Reflex zone massages to the feet were continued at longer intervals, as she was still apt to salivate excessively when under stress. Only a few further treatments were necessary as time went on, and her ataxia disappeared completely.

BACKACHE

A sixty-year-old housewife lay stiffly in bed and had been unable to get up for three days because of acute pain in her right leg and over the coccyx.

The first reflex zone massage was carried out very lightly and, because she was in such pain, it was conducted in the same rhythm as her breathing. Treatment was concentrated on the reflex zones of the lower spine and the pelvic organs on the right side. After fifteen minutes, the pain lessened perceptibly.

The patient was anxious about trying to move at all but was persuaded to try and move her right leg, to find that there was no limitation of movement in either her right leg or her back. She tried walking to the dining room and back and soon fell asleep, considerably relieved and relaxed. Her morning urine, which had been left standing undisturbed for some time, was found to contain a heavy reddish sediment. The day after that, she was able to resume her normal household activities unaided.

BEDWETTING

An eight-year-old child wet the bed every night. There was a distinct visible swelling over the bladder zone on his feet, which was also painful when touched. It was found on physical examination that the reflex zones of the head were even more painful when touched than those of the pelvic areas. After the child had had four treatments, the family moved to another town, but reported eight months later that the child had not wet his bed again after receiving the second treatment.

BILIARY COLIC

During the course of a severe infection, a patient suffered a sudden attack of biliary colic, of which there had been no warning. The reflex zone therapist who was summoned applied firm pressure to the reflex zone of the gallbladder on both dorsal and plantar aspects of the foot, and after about ten seconds, the pain was relieved. The patient suffered no side effects from this treatment.

BRONCHIAL ASTHMA

A sales manager, aged fifty-nine, came to the practice in desolation from severe asthma. A very gentle initial assessment revealed that almost all of his reflex zones were extremely painful. The first treatment provoked a flulike reaction, along with large quantities of dense, smelly mucus from his nose and throat. In the second treatment, a gentle touch of the adrenal zone provoked coughing fits that limited his ability to breathe, again accompanied by large quantities of mucus. But by the fourth treatment, the patient had improved enough to be able to return to work, his breathing became calmer and deeper, and the mucus flowed more easily.

The patient began extending his walks and for the first time in years was able to walk for up to three hours without feeling short of breath. Aside from his twenty-five-year history of asthma, he also suffered from a mild form of diabetes, but a blood sugar test taken after his ninth treatment showed normal levels. After twelve treatments over the course of seven weeks, the patient no longer needed asthma medicine and even left the psychologically important inhaler at home.

BRONCHITIS

A five-year-old girl had suffered from bronchitis since infancy. Most of the time she breathed with her mouth open, and her sinuses were troublesome. Her sleep was disturbed, and she had no appetite.

The reflex zones of her feet were treated with great care, since the child would cry at the slightest touch. After the second treatment, she slept uninterruptedly through the night and was noticeably more cheerful and communicative in the morning. For no apparent reason she developed a runny nose, which stopped after five days, but there was no other sign of a cold. She was now able to bear more pressure on the reflex zones, and over time her pale, crying manner gradually gave way to an impression of health and rosiness. Ten weeks later, she had a medical examination, at which it was found that her nasal polyps had disappeared and that her tonsils were no longer enlarged or inflamed.

BUERGER'S DISEASE

A sixty-seven-year-old engineer who smoked forty cigarettes daily, was unable to walk for a distance of more than fifty yards without having to take a long rest. Before the therapist agreed to start a course of reflex zone massage, he was asked to stop smoking completely, which he agreed to do.

Initially, all the reflex zones of the feet were painful on palpation. It was only after eight treatments that the pain began to be concentrated in the reflex zones of the respiratory tract, the heart, and the pelvic organs. From the second treatment onward he began to produce copious amounts of unusually colored sputum, and this persisted undiminished for six weeks. After he had had sixteen treatments, the patient was able to walk for up to three hours without pain and without having to stop for a rest. He remained a nonsmoker.

CERVICAL SYNDROME

About ten years before she came to the clinic, a fifty-seven-year-old house-wife had needed an upper denture. Two years after that she began to suffer from increasing disability in the cervical spine. X-rays revealed no abnormality, and she did not respond to any tablets, injections, or the heat treatment that had been recommended.

Her first reflex zone massage resulted in a sharp piercing pain in the reflex zone of the rear molar teeth on the left. After two intensive treatments, the left side of the woman's face became extremely painful, red, and swollen. X-rays of the jaw showed that a large piece of the root of the tooth was still present, which required surgery for its removal. Following the extraction the patient suffered no further pain or disability in her neck or cervical spine.

CHRONIC CONSTIPATION

A seventy-one-year-old woman, who was thin and haggard looking, had been having mudpacks applied in an attempt to relieve the pain she felt in her hip but with no effect. On questioning, it was found that she had suffered from constipation for some years.

The tissues of both her feet were atonic and presented a wrinkled and worn appearance. The reflex zones of all her joints and of the alimentary tract were sensitive. She commenced having reflex zone massage of the feet, and after five treatments, the pain in her hip lessened, but her irregular bowel habits persisted. However, the skin of her feet began to improve from one treatment to another, regaining some elasticity while the tissues recovered some tone. The white coat on her tongue began to disappear. At this time she began to break out into nightly sweats, which had a strong odor, and for some days she had a rash of pimples all over her skin. From the eleventh treatment onward her bowel habits became more regular, although she had a lot of flatulence with an offensive smell, and her stools were hard and dark brown.

After thirty treatments, her bowel habits had become quite normal, and she presented an altogether fresher and livelier appearance.

CIRCULATORY DISTURBANCE AFTER JOINT REPLACEMENT

A seventy-five-year-old patient had had two hips replaced within a period of eighteen months. He complained of severe circulatory disturbance in the veins of the right calf and pain and limitation of movement in the right leg.

He was skeptical and anxious at the beginning of the treatment course, fearing that reflex zone massage might worsen his condition. Cautious examination of his feet revealed that reflex zones of all the joints and the spine were painful, and that the reflex zone of the left kidney could hardly be touched. The results of the first treatment were encouraging, as his legs felt warm and relaxed that whole night. However, the patient had to pass urine six times during the night. After only a few massages he was able to take longer walks, and found that walking on hard pavements did not worry him, as it had previously. After six weeks he was able to take his first walk up a mountain incline, to his great delight.

CIRCULATORY DISTURBANCE OF THE HEAD

A fifty-four-year-old sales representative had been receiving medical treatment for many years for a circulatory disorder and had had several thromboses. Since the summer of 1972, his most disturbing symptoms had been headaches and fainting fits, though more recently he had been having attacks of weakness and was no longer able to work. While in the hospital, he had an EEG, which showed evidence of some abnormality in the left upper cerebrum, but it was uncertain whether this was due to early cerebral hemorrhage or to a brain tumor.

The first reflex zone massage had to be carried out with extreme care, since all the reflex zones were very painful. After the third treatment, the sensation of pressure in his head was alleviated, and the painful reflex zones were limited to those of the head, heart, and pelvic region. With continuing treatment, the intervals between his attacks grew longer. An EEG was repeated three months later and was normal. Since then, the patient has been free of all his complaints.

In some astonishment the patient remarked that his toes were also now quite free from pain and that for the first time in thirty years he did not have to have special shoes made to accommodate his previously painful toes.

CONSTIPATION AND CRYING

A five-year-old child would sleep only in a lighted room, woke frequently during the night, and would cry for hours on end without anyone knowing why he was so distressed. He was reserved in nature and found it difficult to communicate or play with other children. Unless he was given laxatives, he had no bowel movements.

The boy's big toe was markedly swollen on the plantar surface. There were painful reflex zones corresponding to the solar plexus and the ascending colon. He came for reflex zone massage twice a week. After he had had ten treatments, he had changed into a playful youngster, was able to sleep at night without needing the light on, and had a normal bowel movement daily. No further laxatives were needed. From discussions, it appeared that the boy had had multiple vaccinations three years previously, following which his ailments had steadily increased.

CONVULSIONS

When he was about six months old, Oliver, a twin, suffered from his first attack of convulsions. He was investigated extensively in a neurological clinic, but his condition did not improve. The infant lay limply and listlessly on his back, and any attempts to sit him up failed.

Both feet were icy cold, particularly the toes, and the pads on the soles of the big toes were taut and swollen. On the dorsum of the feet over the metatarso-phalangeal joints was a firm and swollen area that was very sensitive to touch. After the first three treatments had been very carefully carried out, the mother said that she felt there was some improvement, in that the child seemed to be trying to respond to his parents' attempts to communicate with him. After the fourth treatment, he was able to hold a sitting position for a short while, and did not immediately collapse. While he was in a sitting position, it was noticed that the left half of his rib cage was underdeveloped.

The baby's feet became perceptibly warmer with each treatment, and he started to move them about more. He also began to make efforts to crawl. After twelve treatments, it was possible to communicate almost normally with Oliver. However, the left side of his ribcage continued to sag.

Three months elapsed before he was given a further course of reflex zone massage. He now tended to fall to one side when trying to walk. There had, in the meantime, been a great improvement in the condition of the reflex zones of his feet, and the only ones that were found to be marginally abnormal were those of the head and lower spine, which improved after a further eight treatments. His walking became normal, and he is now indistinguishable from his twin.

DISTURBANCE OF TASTE

The forty-three-year-old wife of a winegrower came for treatment. Disconsolately she recounted that for the past eight months all that she had eaten and drunk had tasted of vinegar. Treatment by a variety of specialists had brought about no improvement.

Palpation of the feet revealed painful zones of the head, neck, lymph vessels, and upper abdomen. After the third treatment, she noticed that from time to time she had a different perception of taste. After ten treatments, she arrived to say that she had eaten six pieces of birthday cake to celebrate having recovered her sense of taste and that it had tasted "even better" than it had before. A total of sixteen treatments was given, and her condition did not recur.

DYSMENORRHEA

A thirty-eight-year-old woman complained of severe pain preceding and during her menstrual periods. Her cycles were irregular and accompanied by depression.

Her feet were visibly gray, and the tissues were atonic. There were calluses over the thyroid and diaphragm reflex zones, and there was a hard, horny area of skin about 0.6 mm thick on each heel, over the reflex zones of the pelvic organs. There was a brown liver spot about the size of a pea over the reflex zone of the sacrum.

Her feet were cool to the touch, and were generally painful when handled with light pressure. The first two treatments lasted only for ten minutes each, as the patient very quickly showed signs of overdose. On the third visit, she arrived feeling surprisingly well and informed me that she had been sleeping well—soundly and dreamlessly. Her foot was now normal to the touch, and the pain she felt during massage of the reflex zones of the pelvic organs and endocrine system—which had been unbearable—had diminished somewhat.

After the sixth treatment, she began to menstruate. Her period was not accompanied by any of the symptoms that had troubled her previously, and there was no swelling or feeling of tension in her breasts. During her period, the patient was given a light and gentle massage to the reflex zones of the genitals. After menstruation had ceased, she suffered a malodorous vaginal discharge, which persisted until the next ovulation. After this she felt better than she had for a long while, but was advised to take regular Sitz baths to completely stabilize her condition.[1]

EARACHE

When he was eighteen years old, a massage therapist of thirty-seven had developed pyelonephritis and hematuria. He had also suffered from angina when he was young. For the past six months, he had been having sensations of pressure and tension in both ears, which were almost painful. He was found on medical examination to have cochlear degeneration, which might have been caused by environmental factors such as noise, exhaust fumes, or something similar. The damage was considered to be irreparable and likely to worsen with age. No form of therapy was thought likely to be effective, so none had been recommended.

Palpation of the feet showed painful reflex zones of the tonsils, upper lymphatics, both kidneys, and the pelvic organs. After the first treatment, the symptoms in his ears disappeared spontaneously, and they have not recurred. (He certainly had strong regenerative capacities, otherwise such a quick result would not have been possible.)

FACIAL NEURALGIA

A forty-three-year-old housewife came for therapy as she had been suffering from facial neuralgia for many years. Painful reflex zones of the sinuses, the left ear, and the bronchi were found on her feet. Between the fourth and fifth toes of the left foot, she had athlete's foot, which she was treating with local applications of an antifungal product. Every time she stopped treatment, the infection recurred a few days later. The first three treatments resulted only in her feeling a sense of general relaxation and sleeping more deeply. After the fourth treatment, she abruptly developed a feverish, flulike illness, with almost purulent mucus secretions from the nose and throat. The patient had never before experienced such a violent illness. On the advice of her doctor, she allowed the fever to run its course naturally without taking any fever-reducing medications. When she recovered, she was no longer troubled with neuralgia, and the athlete's foot healed spontaneously shortly thereafter.

FROZEN SHOULDER

A farmer, who was sixty-one years of age, had suffered from a "frozen" shoulder for eighteen months. A variety of treatments, injections, and thirty massages to the affected area combined with hot mudpacks had brought him no relief.

There was a conspicuous hallux valgus on both feet. The reflex zones of the spine, the shoulder girdle, the liver, and both kidneys were sensitive to pressure. He began to be able to move his shoulder more freely after four treatments. He then suffered an offensive diarrhea for twenty-four hours. After fifteen treatments, his symptoms disappeared completely, and today, three years later, he is able to carry out all the work on his farm without limitation of movement in his shoulder or arm.

GASTRITIS

A notary, aged forty-nine years, had suffered for many years from gastritis, which was accompanied by heartburn and attacks of acidic belching. From an examination of his feet it was seen that the reflex zones of the upper abdomen, the small intestine, the rectum, and the anus were sensitive. A scar was discovered at the reflex zone of the pylorus, though the patient had no memory of an event that could have given rise to such a scar.

The scar was treated by an injection of procaine (Huneke's neural therapy), and soon after this the patient experienced a feeling of warmth and relaxation over the whole of his upper abdomen. As the patient's symptoms disappeared completely after this treatment, and he was kept busy at his office, it was a year before he came for another treatment, this time for an injury that he had sustained at sports practice. There had been no recurrence of his abdominal discomfort during this year.

HEMORRHOIDS

An office worker, fifty-three years old, had for months been using suppositories and ointments in an attempt to relieve her itching and bleeding piles. Before undergoing surgery, she wanted to try reflex zone massage of the feet to see whether it offered her any relief.

On visual examination, the reflex zones around the inner malleoli (which correspond to the true pelvis) were taut and swollen, and the skin there was friable and blue/gray in color. On palpation the reflex zones of the small and large intestine and the base of the spine were distinctly abnormal. During the first four massages, the taut area over the ankles was not touched, as the woman was naturally worried about the possibility of infection here. In place of this, the corresponding reflex zones in the wrists were massaged thoroughly, after which the dark discoloration and swelling around the ankles noticeably subsided, and these areas could subsequently be included in the treatment of her feet.

The nightly itch eased, and her bowels were functioning without pain or blood loss. After a series of twenty treatments, the patient again visited her doctor, who decided that surgery was now unnecessary. The patient noticed and commented on the fact that her thighs and buttocks were no longer cold, and that she was able to walk more easily.

HEADACHE

An eleven-year-old girl had suffered from left-sided headaches since her younger sister had been born when she was five years old. Initially these headaches had occurred every six to eight weeks, but she was now having them every ten days.

On examination of the girl's feet, the reflex zones of the left side of the head were abnormal, and those of the urinary system, the lumbosacral spine, and the genital tract were also painful. After the third reflex zone massage, her headaches became less intense, and after the seventh massage, it was seen that her cheeks were rosier. There followed a long interval in the treatment sessions while the family was away on holiday. During this time she had a vague feeling of being unwell at about three weekly intervals. After some months, she had a further six treatments, and for the last two years she has been a normal, healthy child. It is likely that the intensive attention also contributed to the therapy.

HEART AILMENT

An engineer, fifty-five years old, had received reflex zone massage of the feet at various times in the past. In addition to a backache, he now complained of a deterioration of the heart condition from which he had suffered for the past eight years, and which had not improved with the drug therapy he had been prescribed. He had symptoms of ataxia and said that he felt anxious and uncertain while driving his car.

Physical examination of the feet showed negligible abnormality in the reflex zone of the heart. The reflex zones of the liver, gallbladder, diaphragm, stomach, small intestine, and shoulder girdle were more sensitive to pressure. The first treatment resulted in a release of tension in the muscles of the back and shoulder girdle, and the patient stated that he felt able to breathe more easily. During a series of ten treatments, he suffered from excessive flatulence, but his bowel action returned to normal. He was advised to take a sauna bath once a week, which he does, and for the last two years, he has been free of all symptoms.

HICCUPS

An office worker of fifty-two years of age who was considerably overworked developed hiccups that persisted for six hours. When the office closed, he came for treatment, feeling very depressed. Constant, light pressure for two minutes on the reflex zone of the diaphragm (which relates to breathing as well as the autonomic nervous system) was sufficient to stop the hiccups.

HYDROCEPHALUS

A fifteen-month-old baby was brought from a local nursery for treatment. When she was not sleeping, eating, or crying, she lay apathetically in her cot. She was unable to sit, stand up, or walk, and she did not talk. When she was awake, she moved her head from side to side in a continuous rocking movement. As soon as her head stopped moving, she would cry out. Medical opinion stated that she was mentally retarded.

Upon examination, her big toes were found to be swollen, taut, and tense. After the first reflex zone massage, she spontaneously stopped rocking her head from side to side, and she seemed to be calmer. After the second treatment, to the astonishment of her mother and the therapist, she pulled herself into a sitting position with great effort. She attempted to stand after the third treatment. From the seventh treatment onward, she behaved in a normal fashion for her age.

When treatment was started on this child, her head circumference was 46.5 cm. This remained the same while she grew in body length from 24.5 inches to 29 inches, by which time the relationship between the circumference of her head and her body length was evidently normal.

After two years—the child is now a little more than three years old—the impression that she gives is that she is a normal toddler. Her physical development is retarded by about four months, and arrangements have been made for her to have a further series of reflex zone massages to her feet.

Please note that such surprising results cannot be replicated everywhere. Each healing process depends not only on the chosen therapy and quality of the therapist but also on the regenerative powers of the patient, as well as other factors.

HYPERTENSION

A fifty-eight-year-old textile merchant was sixty pounds overweight, and complained of sensations of pressure in his head, fainting, restless sleep, and nervousness, and said that he had little appetite for food. His blood pressure was 195/95.

On examination, the tissues of his feet were generally rough and gray, and the reflex zones of the upper abdomen and head were very sensitive to touch. He was considerably distressed by the pain that he experienced during the first treatment and wanted time to consider whether or not he would return for a second treatment. He returned three days later in some dudgeon, as he had been considerably troubled by diarrhea and flatulence during that time. In the meantime, the reflex zones had become a little less painful. His treatment continued, and after the fifth massage, the man came to terms with this unusual method of treatment. He told friends and acquaintances that his symptoms had been relieved and that he now felt very well.

He allowed himself to be persuaded that his sumptuous evening meals were harming rather than helping him, and he managed to lose forty-five pounds in four months. Eighteen months later, he had a medical examination, at which it was found that his blood pressure and liver function tests had returned to normal.

HYPERTHYROIDISM

A thirty-nine-year-old businesswoman, the mother of four lively children, complained of increasing hyperthyroidism. She was losing weight rapidly, cried at the least provocation, and could not sleep at night.

Her first reflex zone massage was concluded after ten minutes, since the patient began to cry violently and was beginning to shiver. A thorough palpation of the reflex zones was only possible at the second treatment and was carried out lightly and delicately. This showed abnormal reflex zones of the entire endocrine system, as well as of the solar plexus and head.

The following treatments consisted predominantly of soothing, stroking movements. From the fifth treatment, her condition began to stabilize, and she became less agitated. After the eighth treatment she menstruated normally, without pain, and with relatively little blood loss. Shortly afterwards the feeling that she had previously had of having a lump in her throat began to disappear, along with the difficulties in swallowing that had plagued her. She had gained thirteen pounds after sixteen treatments, and said that she felt as though she was once more in control of her life.

HYPOTENSION

A thirty-four-year-old businesswoman, slightly built and anxious, came for treatment for low blood pressure—90/65. She explained that she did not feel that there was anything "organically" wrong but that she felt like a "wilting house plant."

All the reflex zones from the heel to the toes were painful for the first three massages. At the beginning of the fourth treatment the patient burst into tears, and was encouraged to cry freely. This release of tension was evident on the feet immediately—the reflex zone of the solar plexus (which is the same as that of the diaphragm) was no longer painful, and much to the astonishment of both patient and practitioner, neither were any of the other reflex zones. After fourteen treatments, her condition had improved so much that she was able to resume work feeling restored. Her blood pressure stabilized at 120/90, and her sleep became deep and restful.

IMPAIRED VISION

An active, alert, retired woman of seventy-two years had suffered severe impairment of her vision over the past three months, for no apparent cause. Since she did not wish to go into an old people's home, she had tried every available means of treatment to restore her sight but had not been helped by any of them. She decided that she would try a course of reflex zone massage as a last resort.

On palpation the reflex zones of the eyes, kidneys, and bladder were very painful. Between the second and third toes, she had athlete's foot, which was very irritating and had persisted for four months, and she had no explanation as to its cause.

After the second treatment, the patient began to sleep more soundly at night and did not have to get up to empty her bladder two to four times during the night as had previously been the case.

At the third treatment, she said that the dark veil that had lain in front of her eyes had lightened and that she was now able to distinguish colors again. After the fourth treatment, she was able to read her Bible. Over the next four years, she came for four additional series of treatments—none of which were for her poor sight but for some other ailments that commonly occur in old age. Because of her strong regenerative powers, six to eight sessions sufficed for each treatment series.

INFECTED FOCUS IN A TOOTH

A professional sportsman, aged twenty-one, had had severe pain in his lower back for several weeks. He had tried various methods of treatment, none of which brought him any relief. He was not able to participate in any sporting activity unless he had previously had injections of painkillers.

The reflex zones of the lower half of the spine were very sensitive on palpation, and so, surprisingly, were the reflex zones of the head. After the third treatment, he developed a fever and a very severe toothache. The dentist found an infected focus in his apparently healthy teeth; after the tooth was extracted, the young man's backache disappeared.

INFECTIOUS HEPATITIS

A therapist sent in this account of her own illness: "Two years ago I became acutely ill with viral hepatitis. For weeks beforehand, I had noticed that there was pain over the areas of my feet that represented the liver, stomach, and solar plexus while standing, but which became concentrated in one small area in the reflex zone of the liver until the outbreak of the illness. A sharply defined bluish area of about 1 cm in diameter was also plainly visible over this point.

During my stay in the hospital, I frequently worked on the sensitive reflex zones of the upper abdomen and spleen. I could hardly touch the reflex zone of the liver. As my condition improved, the reflex zone of the liver became less painful to palpation, and the bluish point disappeared but remains today, barely visible, as a pale yellow discoloration of the skin."

INTERMITTENT CLAUDICATION

A forty-eight-year-old industrial consultant came for treatment and was found to have greatly swollen legs, in which he complained of severe cramplike pains. His hearing, vision, and memory had deteriorated, and he complained of circulatory problems and backache as well. There were hard calluses on both heels around the area corresponding to the pelvic organs and also on the base of the toe joints, corresponding to the neck region. Palpation verified visual observation, as all the reflex zones of the pelvis, the head, and the shoulder girdle were sensitive. Results showed themselves after the first treatment in a relaxation of tension in the entire musculature of the back and legs.

This man required fifteen treatments before he was once more without pain and able to return to work. The nightly pacing about his room, due to cramps in the legs and tension and excessive warmth of the feet, ceased as the pain was relieved, and he was visibly restored to health.

IRRITABLE BLADDER

A lively and busy seamstress of fifty years of age had suffered from an irritable bladder for the past three years. No organic disorder was found during several medical examinations. On her feet, the reflex zones of the bladder, the solar plexus, the lumbo-sacral spine, and—more than any other—the reflex zone of the pharynx, were painful. After the first treatment, she found that she only needed to empty her bladder every three hours, but she developed a heavy cold that lasted for two days and then disappeared.

Six reflex zone massages to the feet were all that were needed by this patient before she was relieved of all her symptoms. A year later she remains well.

KIDNEY STONES

A mechanical engineer, fifty-four years old, had previously had surgery to remove a kidney stone. When he was discovered to have a stone forming in his kidney two years later, he decided to try a series of reflex zone massages to the feet before undergoing further surgery.

The findings were of strong pain in the reflex zones of the left kidney and the lower spine. After two intensive treatments, the patient stated that the nature of his pain had changed, in that it was now lower down and tracking further downward toward his bladder. He deduced that the stone was descending down the ureter. After eleven days, two stones entered the bladder, and he had colicky pain and hematuria. Two days later, the stones were passed in the urine and were found on examination to be oxalate stones.

MIGRAINE

A forty-two-year-old patient complained of almost daily attacks of migraine headache, which he had been having with increasing severity for the past ten years. Because of his frequent absences from work, he was about to lose his position.

On palpation, the reflex zones of the head, liver, stomach, and lymphatic system were sensitive. The feet were treated at intervals of three days. After the seventh treatment, the man was no longer in need of the usual medications for his headaches, and his headaches did not recur even at times of great stress at work. He was given, in all, fourteen massages to the reflex zones of the feet and noted with some astonishment that his circulation had greatly improved, even though he was no longer taking any drugs for this either.

OSTEOARTHRITIS

A hotelier of sixty-eight years of age came for treatment because of severe pain in all her large joints. She was hardly capable of dressing and undressing herself and had tried several remedies but gained no relief from them.

Examination of the feet showed that the reflex zones of the kidneys and the entire alimentary tract were more sensitive to touch than were those of the large joints. After five treatments, her reactions took the form of frequent and fetid stools and urine, but her joints were becoming more free in their movement. She was given twelve treatments in all and reported a year later that she had remained well. The following autumn, she returned for two prophylactic treatments.

PARALYTIC ILEUS

Following surgery for removal of a kidney stone, a patient developed a paralytic ileus. Enemas and other conventional treatments did not bring about any improvement, and the condition of the patient worsened rapidly.

Reflex zone massage of the feet was carried out by a doctor friend who was, by chance, visiting the patient at that time. Within a very few minutes of treatment, some bowel sounds were heard. The prompt effectiveness of this treatment reminded both the doctor and the patient of the "lightning phenomenon" described by Huneke.

PROSTATITIS WITH DIFFICULT URINATION

A participant at one of our courses learned from his massage partner that his reflex zone of the prostate gland was particularly sensitive. At that time, he was not aware of any symptoms, but eight weeks later, he developed painful prostatitis and had difficulty passing urine. A medical examination found the prostate gland to be hypertrophied.

The symptoms were alleviated after ten reflex zone massages to his feet. He no longer had urinary frequency during the night, and his urinary stream was strong. A medical examination confirmed that the prostate gland was normal.

PYLORIC STENOSIS

A four-month-old boy was due to have surgery in two weeks for pyloric stenosis. A reflex zone therapist asked if she could see the feet of the baby.

She found on palpation that there was a painful response on the precise area of the reflex zone of the stomach and solar plexus. The next day she was told that, for the first time, the infant been able to nurse without vomiting afterward. He was given two further treatments, and his grandmother was shown how to massage the sensitive zones carefully and asked to do so each evening.

Six months later, the baby was again brought for a visit. As his condition had improved so markedly, it had not been necessary for him to have the operation that had been planned.

PYRETIC INFECTION

A quiet, thin, sensitive child of seven had suffered for more than a year from chronic sniffles, a feeling of heaviness in his head, general lassitude, and bouts of fever. He had to be protected from inclement weather or he would develop a fever the following day and have to be put to bed. He was not making any progress at school.

Examination of the feet showed the reflex zones to the bronchi, sinuses, kidneys, and spleen to be very painful. After the third and fourth treatments, his previously watery catarrh became yolk colored, and he developed a slight cough. Following the sixth reflex zone massage of his feet, the boy reported with amazement that he was able to smell things again and that the sense of pressure in his head was not so great.

He had, in all, ten treatments, each given quite precisely up to the level of his pain threshold. When he was caught in the rain one day, he suffered no relapse, and eighteen months later the boy gives the impression of being bright and lively.

RECTAL PROLAPSE

An eighty-three-year-old woman had suffered from a rectal prolapse since the birth of her last child(!).

Examination of the feet revealed that all the reflex zones of the entire pelvic area were abnormal. After the first treatment, the patient said she no longer experienced a sensation of pressure around her anus, and four additional treatments confirmed this spontaneous resolution of her ailment, which surely also had much to do with her innate regenerative powers.

SCIATICA

A carpenter, aged forty-six, had not been able to work for six weeks because of sciatica. Heat treatments, injections, and salves had brought him no relief. He came for treatment limping and in obvious pain.

The reflex zones of the true pelvis, the lower spine, and particularly those of the kidneys were very painful when touched. This seemed strange, as the man said his urine was clear and micturition caused him no problems. After the first reflex zone massage, he was able to walk a little more easily, and after the third treatment, he was free of pain when walking. After four treatments, he was able to return to work. However, his urine was now dark and cloudy and gave off a strong odor. After eight treatments, his urine returned to a normal color, volume, and odor, and his sciatic pain finally disappeared completely, while he was walking and at rest. The patient took seriously the advice to drink more liquids.

SLIPPED DISC

A farmer, aged thirty-eight and the mother of three children, suffered from a slipped disc in the lumbar area of her spine and spent months in unsuccessful treatments, including massages, baths, injections, and sessions with a chiropractor. She was not able to work in the field or to drive her tractor.

The visual assessment of her feet showed that the zones of the upper and lower spine were marked by calluses, extending into the tissue of the lumbar zone. Palpation revealed very painful kidney and genital zones, especially on the right foot. In the night following the first treatment, the woman suffered from cramplike pains in the lower part of her back, which slowly decreased after she urinated five times over the course of two hours. It is likely that some problems in the kidney, perhaps small stones, were released in this way—not a rare reaction to the treatment of the zones of the feet. The third treatment provoked a strong increase in a brown vaginal secretion that stopped after the next menstruation.

After the eighth treatment, the reflex zones were almost completely free of pain, at which point the woman was shown some posture correction tips recommended by the Alexander Technique,[2] which she could use in the course of her daily tasks. By harvest time, she was able to work fully, and two years later, the foot no longer showed any calluses, even though the woman never went to a podiatrist.

TOOTH EXTRACTION

A thirty-seven-year-old saleswoman had a tooth extracted from her upper jaw. As a result, a sinus had formed between the maxilla and the nose. When breathing in, she was aware of a passage of air from the mouth to the nose through this sinus. She had been told by the dentist that it would heal in time without surgery.

She was given ten reflex zone treatments to see what effect they had.

At the end of this course of treatment, the sinus had healed completely, and she was free of pain and discomfort. In addition to the head zones, the zones of the true pelvis had also been treated.

TORTICOLLIS

Overnight a fifty-five-year-old car salesman developed an extremely painful and stiff neck. It was only with great difficulty that he was able to move his head, neck, or shoulder.

He was given reflex zone massage for ten-minute periods at a time in his home. This consisted largely of a careful but sustained rotation of the basal joint of the big toe, which brought about a reflex relaxation of the musculature of the neck. The immobility and acute pain resolved spontaneously and there was no recurrence of it. That evening he was able to sell three cars!

TREATMENT FOLLOWING A FALL FROM A HORSE

A manufacturer of thirty-nine, who was a passionate rider, fell from his horse and suffered extensive bruising over the upper part of his spine and left shoulder. He was taken by a friend to the hospital where several X-rays were taken, which showed no fractures. The man was then brought for reflex zone massage of his feet. His pain was relieved within thirty minutes, and the man was able to walk away unaided after the treatment was over. He was given a further three massages to promote healing of the bruised tissues. After that, he registered for the next tournament.

UNDESCENDED TESTES

A twelve-year-old boy, whose teacher complained of his lack of concentration and his apathy, had not, so far, responded to any of the tonics prescribed for him. Physical examination of the feet showed disturbed circulation in the reflex zones of the genital area, the head, the adrenal glands, and the stomach. A medical examination was made, and he was diagnosed with an undescended testicle.

Over the course of ten reflex zone massages, the boy's testes descended to a normal position. He subsequently found his schoolwork much easier to attend to and, a year later, was one of the best pupils in the class.

VARICOSE VEINS

A thirty-six-year-old waitress complained of marked congestion and pain in the veins of her legs. On the right shin, there was a hot and somewhat reddened area. As she had no varicose veins on her feet and ankles, it was possible to palpate the reflex zones of her feet. The reflex zones of the pelvic organs (particularly those of the rectum and anus), the liver, the small intestine, and the spleen were very painful.

After the first treatment, the patient reported that she experienced a "lightening" of the pain in her legs for about six hours. The red area on her shin was treated by massaging the corresponding area on the forearm of the same side. Although very light pressure had been applied, a hematoma developed on the forearm over this area, but the angry red area on the shin disappeared.

Over the course of fourteen reflex zone massages, the bones of the woman's ankles became visible once more as the ankles slimmed down, and the reflex zones of this area were no longer painful. The patient remarked that following the third treatment, her urinary output had increased markedly, and that her menstrual irregularities were no longer evident. In addition to treatment, she had also adjusted her diet.

SUMMARY

The case histories reviewed on the preceding pages indicate a number of important therapeutic observations:

- It is not only the diagnosis of the illness that affects the result of treatment but also the quality of the patient's inner regenerative capacity (what Paracelsus termed the "Inner Doctor").
- Both the technical and human qualities of the therapist influence the result of therapy.
- The sooner a patient is ready to make changes in his or her lifestyle, the more lasting the result of treatment is likely to be.

PART FOUR

INDICATIONS

24

Using Treatment Indications

The following guidelines for treatment have been drawn up after many years of clinical practice and experience in reflex zone therapy. However, they cannot be regarded as any more than an orientation to the general pattern that treatment should follow.

Far more important than the prescriptions printed here is the practitioner's grasp of the complexity of each patient's individual disease background and the close observation of reactions in every single patient as soon as they occur.

These understandings depend in every case on thorough visual and physical examinations of the feet during the first reflex zone massage. From these initial exams, a composite picture is developed. While the first observations form a guideline for the treatment that follows, it must constantly be borne in mind that the reactions that subsequently manifest in the patient can bring about modification of the findings and consequent treatment pattern. Therapists who treat the same zones every time have failed to recognize that health and illness are dynamic processes that continue to evolve constantly.

Visual observation provides the practitioner with the first indication of abnormal reflex zones on the feet. In order to have validity, however, such visual observations must always be confirmed by physical palpation.

Painful reflex zones can arise because of a disease that is still insignificant and not yet clinically detectable, because of weakness or overtaxation of an organ, or as the result of acute or chronic disorders. Even where zones are not felt as painful, the autonomic nervous system often gives clear indications of stress on the zones (sweaty hands, change in breathing, pulse rate, facial color, and so forth).

Reflex zones that are painful during the first massage are divided into two groups:

1. The symptomatic zones, in which treatment will be concentrated initially.
2. The background zones, the discovery of which will illuminate the causes and consequences of the presenting symptoms, accurately indicating those tissues, organs, or systems that are under stress.

Background zones can be zones where a patient's weakness or disability originated and/or zones that have been handicapped by the disease process, as happens to the reflex zone of the solar plexus, for instance, when pain is present, or to the reflex zones of the lymphatic system during infections.

The following lists of symptomatic and background zones must be tested during each patient's first reflex zone massage. Such testing will prove its aptness and veracity and will ensure that your treatment departs from a static, prescribed form and brings to life a creative skill. These guidelines for treatment will then be what they are intended to be: a signpost, which is not the pathway itself, but which points the direction.

Naturally, the schematic presentation of this mixed table cannot comprehend the individual variations on all feet. This comprehension can only be attained by constant, vigilant observation and sensitive palpation.

Indications for
Reflex Zone Therapy

ALLERGY, ECZEMA

SZ: (Symptomatic Zones) Endocrine system, lymphatic system.

BZ: (Background Zones): Liver and gallbladder, small intestine, large intestine, kidneys, spleen, solar plexus; localized infection.

Treatment Notes: Use balancing grips and pay attention to diet!

APOPLEXY

SZ: All the organs of the head (particularly the big toe, which is the site of cerebral catastrophe reflected on the reflex zones of the feet), solar plexus. Be careful with initial dosage on the head.

BZ: Solar plexus, kidneys, heart, genitals, intestine, cervical spine, neck, and spleen.

Treatment Notes: Use balancing grips.

ARM INJURIES

SZ: Cervical spine, shoulder girdle, shoulder joint, upper arm and elbow, teeth.

BZ: Intestines, teeth, kidneys, lumbar spine.

Treatment Notes: Corollary areas to be treated include the same area on the opposite arm, and an "energetically related area"—the corresponding area of the leg on the same side as the injured arm.

ARTHRITIS, ARTHROSES

SZ: All joints, particularly those that are most affected; spine. Begin gently and softly!

BZ: Small intestine, large intestine, stomach, liver and gallbladder, lymphatic system—both of the upper body and of the pelvis; kidneys, adrenal glands, solar plexus, spleen, sinuses, teeth, and scars.

Treatment Notes: Use balancing grips. Counsel patient regarding a change in diet!

AUTONOMIC DYSFUNCTION

SZ: Solar plexus, head.

BZ: Heart, endocrine system (particularly the pituitary gland and the genitals) liver, intestines, kidneys, spine, shoulder girdle, sternum, and spleen.

Treatment Notes: Many balancing grips. Pay attention to calm breathing during treatment and graduate dosage with care.

BEDWETTING

SZ: Urinary tract, genitals, lymphatics of the pelvis and inguinal canal.

BZ: Lower spine, solar plexus, endocrine system.

Treatment Notes: Avoid strong geopathic irritations and unhealthy stimuli in the surroundings. Also treat irritated parents.

BREAST SWELLING AND TENDERNESS

SZ: Breasts and upper lymphatics.

BZ: Shoulder girdle, genitals, solar plexus, pelvic lymphatics, spleen, and teeth.

Treatment Notes: If there is no improvement after the next menstrual period, the patient should be advised to seek medical advice.

BRONCHIAL ASTHMA

SZ: Respiratory tract, throat, upper lymphatics, diaphragm, and sternum.

BZ: Neck, occiput, shoulder girdle; all organs of the digestive tract (particularly the small intestine and the ileocecal valve); the endocrine system (particularly the adrenal glands); the spleen, heart, and spine.

Treatment Notes: Use many balancing grips. When an acute attack threatens, firmly grip the webs between the second and third toes of both feet (lymph areas of head and throat), and massage the solar plexus reflex zone.

BRONCHITIS, BRONCHIECTASIS

SZ: Respiratory tract, throat, upper lymphatics, and diaphragm.

BZ: Small intestine (particularly the ileocecal valve), large intestine, liver and gallbladder, shoulder girdle, solar plexus, spleen, genitals, urinary tract, heart.

CERVICAL SYNDROME

SZ: Cervical spine, neck, shoulder girdle, and head.

BZ: Lower spine, solar plexus, teeth, pelvis.

Treatment Notes: Begin working gently with sedating grips, consider starting with BZs. Check for tissue changes around the 7th cervical vertebra. Work on correction of posture.

CHOLECYSTITIS

SZ: Gallbladder on both plantar and dorsal aspects, liver, and small intestine—particularly the duodenum.

BZ: Right half of the shoulder girdle, solar plexus, large intestine, pancreas, and thoracic spine.

Treatment Notes: Pay attention to diet! Also that which angers and worries the patient.

For colic, use the sedation grip on symptomatic zones and the solar plexus zone. Tone small intestine.

CONCUSSION

SZ: All head zones, particularly the occiput and cervical spine. Work very gently using the sedation grip.

BZ: Solar plexus, heart, upper lymphatics, lower spine, and stomach.

Treatment Notes: With severe stresses it is always helpful to begin by massaging the reflex zones **far** from the symptoms or even to avoid the SZs. Use many balancing grips!

CONSTIPATION

SZ: Large intestine (particularly the sigmoid, rectum, and anus), liver, gallbladder, and small intestine (particularly the ileocecal valve).

BZ: Pelvic lymphatics, lower spine, solar plexus, stomach, pancreas, head, endocrine system.

Treatment Notes: Investigate the dietary habits.[1]

CYSTITIS, IRRITABLE BLADDER

SZ: Bladder, ureter.

BZ: Lower spine, kidneys, pelvic lymphatics, genitals (particularly the prostate in male patients), spleen, solar plexus, pharynx, and larynx.

Treatment Notes: Work gently and with many balancing grips.

DIABETES MELLITUS

SZ: Pancreas. Begin with gentle stimulation!

BZ: Endocrine system, solar plexus (in shock diabetes), small intestine, large intestine, liver and gallbladder, spleen, eyes, and teeth.

Treatment Notes: This is supplementary treatment for patients who control their blood sugar levels by drug administration. Regular assessment of blood sugar levels is necessary, especially in acute infections. Recommend plenty of exercise, fresh air, and a good diet. Use balancing grips.

DIARRHEA

SZ: Small intestine, pylorus, and ileocecal valve. Work to sedate!

BZ: Solar plexus, liver and gallbladder, large intestine, stomach, pancreas, endocrine system, and middle spine.

Treatment Notes: Use balancing grips.

EAR INFECTIONS

SZ: Ears, lymphatics of the throat, and pharynx.

BZ: Teeth and sinuses, upper lymphatics, solar plexus, spleen, appendix, stomach, and digestive tract.

Treatment Notes: For treatment of acute otitis media, begin gently with the sedation grip in the symptomatic zones. Use balancing grips.

EPILEPSY

SZ: Endocrine system, solar plexus, head (with soft sedating grip), and lymphatics.

BZ: Spine, liver and gallbladder, small and large intestines, spleen, scars.

Treatment Notes: Check for existing disturbed fields, and for scars—especially in the head area. Use many balancing grips and recommend classical homeopathy as supplementary therapy.

FRACTURES

SZ: Those zones that correspond to the injured tissues surrounding the fracture, lymphatics, solar plexus.

Treatment Notes: For fractures of the extremities, work on corrolary and energetically related areas with the usual massage grip. Use balancing grips.

GLAUCOMA

SZ: Head, particularly the eyes.

BZ: Cervical spine, sinuses, shoulder girdle, upper lymphatics, teeth and throat, kidneys, pancreas, and solar plexus.

Treatment Notes: Reflex zone therapy should only be used as a supplementary measure. Patients should be under the care of a doctor.

HAYFEVER

SZ: Area of the nose and throat, sinuses. When symptoms are acute, begin by sedating.

BZ: Upper lymphatics, liver, small intestine (particularly the ileocecal valve), large intestine, bronchi, endocrine system, kidneys, and spleen.

Treatment Notes: Use balancing grips. Recommend dietary changes, discuss lactose intolerance.

HEADACHE, MIGRAINE

SZ: Head (particularly the mastoid process), neck, and cervical spine. When acute begin with a sedating grip.

BZ: Shoulder girdle, lymphatics, small and large intestines, stomach, liver and gallbladder (frequently the most distressed), spine, urinary tract, genitals, solar plexus.

Treatment Notes: In women, headaches are often associated with menstrual disorders. Use balancing grips. Posture should be corrected if necessary.

HEART AND CIRCULATORY DISORDERS

SZ: Spleen, heart (start very carefully), left side of the shoulder girdle as far as the indirect reflex zone to the elbow, the sternum (which should be very gently treated immediately after an infarct). Treat the spleen before the heart.

BZ: Diaphragm, upper lymphatics, liver and gallbladder, stomach, small and large intestines, the diaphragm over the area where maximal stimulus is effected (because of the gastrocardial symptom complex); the cervical spine (particularly the seventh cervical vertebra, and by very gently rotating the big toe on its base joint); solar plexus, scars, and teeth.

Treatment Notes: Use balancing grips! This therapy may be used as prophylaxis against infarction or as treatment for recent or past myocardial infarction.

HERNIA

SZ: Inguinal canal (particularly on the medial aspect related to the same body zone on the feet), pelvic lymphatics, and genitals.

BZ: Lower spine, bladder, endocrine system (particularly the pituitary gland), solar plexus.

Treatment Notes: Use plenty of balancing grips. Treatment can also be used postoperatively.

HYPERTENSION AND HYPOTENSION

SZ: Head (begin gently in cases of hypotension), neck, heart, and solar plexus.

BZ: Shoulder girdle, kidneys, genitals, spine, digestive tract, foci (scars and teeth), and endocrine system.

Treatment Notes: Use balancing grips.

JOINT DISORDERS

In addition to massage of the symptomatic reflex zones and the background zones of specific joints, corollary treatment of the joints may be given. For example, if there is pain or disability of the shoulder joint, the opposite shoulder joint can be treated, and if the ankle joint is painful and/or impaired in function, the opposite ankle can be treated. The energetically related joint may also be treated, such that when there is dysfunction of a hip joint, the shoulder joint on the same side of the body is treated. Similarly, the hip joint on the same side of the body is treated when there is dysfunction of the shoulder joint. This allows treatment of knee joints for the elbow joints and vice versa; joints of the hands for joints of the feet and vice versa; and treatment of the same joint on the opposite side of the body. These areas are treated with the customary massage grip. Also treat the zones of the secreting organs (i.e., kidneys, intestines), liver, spleen, and solar plexus. Check teeth and scars for possible fields of disturbances.

LEG INJURIES

SZ: Lower spine, pelvic region, hip and knee joints.

BZ: Pelvic area, intestines, teeth, and sinus region.

Treatment Notes: Corollary areas that can be treated include the corresponding area on the other leg, and the energetically related limb—that is, the arm on the same side of the body as the injured leg.

LYMPHATIC OBSTRUCTION DURING PREGNANCY

SZ: Lymphatics of the pelvis and shoulder girdle, endocrine system.

BZ: Heart, spleen, urinary tract, liver and gallbladder, small intestine, large intestine (particularly the rectum and anus), solar plexus, and spine.

Treatment Notes: The first treatment should be very carefully and accurately dosed starting in the third or fourth month of pregnancy. Do not use in high-risk pregnancies. Use balancing grips.

MENISCUS INJURIES

SZ: Knee joint.

BZ: Lower spine, hip joint, pelvic region, pelvic lymphatics.

Treatment Notes: Use plenty of balancing grips! Since there are six acupuncture meridians that energetically supply the knee, it is also useful to check for distress in the zones of the liver, kidney, pancreas (yin meridians), and bladder, gallbladder, stomach (yang meridians). Check for disturbances from scars and teeth. Treatment may also be applied to the energetically related zones of the opposite knee and the elbow on the same side. May also be used as postoperative treatment.

MENSTRUAL DISORDERS

SZ: Pelvic lymphatics, genitals, and fallopian tubes.

BZ: Endocrine system (particularly the pituitary and thyroid glands), lower spine, solar plexus, pelvic region, intestines, kidneys, and thighs.

Treatment Notes: Use balancing grips. It is helpful to inform your female patients that menstruation may occur either earlier or later than expected, as reflex zone massage sometimes changes the cycle.

PERIPHERAL VASCULAR DISEASE

SZ: Shoulder and hip joints; lymphatics of the pelvis and the shoulder girdle, spine.

BZ: Liver and gallbladder, small and large intestines, heart, solar plexus, endocrine system (particularly the pancreas), scars.

Treatment Notes: Attention should be given to corollary relationships!

PROSTATE DISORDER

SZ: Genitals and pelvic lymphatics.

BZ: Endocrine system, urinary system, lower spine, solar plexus, inguinal canal, throat, and teeth.

Treatment Notes: Check for infections of the teeth, and for scars along the center of the body. This treatment can also be used postoperatively.

RENAL DISEASE

SZ: Kidneys, ureter, and bladder.

BZ: Lower spine, lymphatics of the pelvis and the inguinal region, spleen, heart, digestive tract, endocrine system, and eyes as well as yet unapparent disease, scars or chronic infections of an organ, or devitalized or impacted teeth.

Treatment Notes: For pain, use sedation grips.

RHEUMATISM

SZ: All painful joints, and all painful organs and/or muscles. Begin by working gently with sedating grips.

BZ: Liver, small and large intestines, entire lymphatic system, spine, solar plexus, kidneys, adrenal glands, spleen.

Treatment Notes: Check for disturbances in teeth and for scars. Dietary habits and nutrition should be investigated.

SCAR TREATMENTS

Strongly tone the zones of the foot that correspond to the scars. Massage the solar plexus zone and use balancing grips to harmonize the emotional level. This can be done starting about three weeks following surgery or injury, even on scars in the stomach region and on the head. Use topical scar creams several times a day, both on the scar itself and on its reflex zone on the feet. Scars that have been present for a long time can still be bothersome! Consider if neural therapy is needed in addition.

SCIATICA, LUMBAGO

SZ: Lower spine, sides of abdominal muscles.

BZ: Kidneys, liver, intestines, pelvic lymphatics, genitals, upper and lower spine, solar plexus.

Treatment Notes: Use plenty of balancing grips. Check for scars and/or infected teeth. It may be necessary to correct posture.

SINUSITIS

SZ: All the sinus cavities of the head, and the lymphatics of the face and throat (particularly the tonsils).

BZ: Head, shoulder girdle, bronchi, spleen, small intestine (particularly the ileocecal valve), liver, large intestine, pancreas, urinary system, genitals, solar plexus.

Treatment Notes: If the sinuses are not secreting mucus, work to tone the zones in order to stimulate secretions. Otherwise, begin with sedating grips.

SLEEP DISTURBANCES

SZ: Solar plexus.

BZ: Endocrine system (particularly the adrenal and pituitary glands), heart, spine, liver and gallbladder, small intestine, large intestine, and shoulder girdle.

Treatment Notes: Use many balancing grips. Avoid geopathic irritations as well as radios, television, computers, and digital clocks in the bedroom. It may be necessary to change dietary habits.

STOMACH DISORDERS

SZ: Stomach, cardia, and pylorus. Begin gently.

BZ: Solar plexus, middle spine, small intestine (particularly the duodenum), large intestine, liver and gallbladder, pancreas, endocrine system (particularly the pituitary gland).

Treatment Notes: Use plenty of balancing grips. Check for disturbances from teeth and from scars. Check whether dietary habits and/or lifestyle need modification.

TOOTHACHE

Reflex zone massage is no substitute for the dentist! As a first aid measure, use the sedation grip on the zone that corresponds to the afflicted tooth or teeth. Patients can also treat themselves every 30 to 60 minutes using zones on the hand. Focus on the zones of the excretion organs, and on the spleen, tonsils, and appendix. Use many balancing grips.

In the case of bleeding gums, gently tone all tooth and digestive zones. Bleeding gums may be an indication that a metal which is antipathetic to the body has been used to fill the teeth or as a brace. Such metals should be removed and any subclinical disease should be treated. Nutrition should be improved.

Although the teeth are essential for mastication and speech, they are also related to every organ via the energy fields they share.

TONSILLITIS

SZ: Tonsils, lymphatics of the throat, neck.

BZ: Entire lymphatic system, all head zones, spleen, cervical spine, shoulder girdle, ileocecal valve and appendix, digestive tract, liver, small intestine, heart.

Treatment Notes: Begin by working gently with sedating grips. Use balancing grips on background zones. This therapy can also be effective as postoperative treatment (scar!).

THYROID DISORDERS

SZ: Thyroid gland, throat.

BZ: Endocrine system, (in women particularly the ovaries), shoulder girdle, cervical spine, solar plexus, intestines, heart, lymphatics, and teeth.

Treatment Notes: Commence treatment extremely gently when the patient has hyperthyroidism and use many balancing grips.

VARICOSE VEINS, PHLEBITIS

SZ: Lymphatics of the pelvic region, liver.

BZ: Small intestine, large intestine (particularly the rectum and anus), heart, spleen, diaphragm, and spine.

Treatment Notes: When the varicose veins are far advanced or infected, the corresponding area on the arm (on the same side of the body) should be massaged instead. Thrombophlebitis is a contraindication for reflex zone massage. Check dietary habits (often too acidic).

WORK-RELATED STRESS

SZ: Solar plexus, heart, and sternum.

BZ: Liver, small intestine (particularly the duodenum), spleen, stomach, large intestine, endocrine system, head, spine, and shoulder girdle.

Treatment Notes: Begin with sedating and plenty of balancing grips.

ULCERS OF THE FEET

SZ: Lymphatics of the pelvis.

BZ: Liver, small intestine, large intestine, rectum, anus, urinary tract, and endocrine system (particularly the pancreas). If ulceration is above the inner side of the ankle, add kidneys, liver, spleen, and pancreas.

Treatment Notes: Work collaterally and, if possible, contralaterally. Attention should be given to nutrition.

Notes

CHAPTER 1. THE HISTORY OF REFLEX ZONE THERAPY

1. William H. Fitzgerald and Edwin F. Bowers, *Zone Therapy: Relieving Pain at Home* (Pomeroy: WA: Health Research Books, 1994).
2. Ibid.
3. Ingham, *Stories the Feet Can Tell thru Reflexology.*

CHAPTER 2. THE ZONE GRID

1. Hanne Marquardt, *Praktisches Lehrbuch des Reflexzonentherapie am Fuß* (Stuttgart: Hippokrates, 2001).

CHAPTER 3. THE CONCEPT OF REFLEX ZONES

1. H. Helmrich, *Kompendium der Bindegewebsmassage* [Compendium of Connective Tissue Massage] (Heidelberg: Karl F. Haug Verlag, 1994).
2. W. Pschyrembel, *Klinisches Wörterbuch* [Clinical Dictionary] (Berlin: Verlag Walter de Gruyler, 1993).

CHAPTER 5. BURDENED REFLEX ZONES OF THE FOOT

1. Eunice D. Ingham, *Stories the Feet Can Tell thru Reflexology* and *Stories the Feet Have Told thru Reflexology* (St. Petersburg: FL: Ingham Publishing, 1984).

CHAPTER 10. THE GRIP SEQUENCE

1. Sebastian Kneipp, *Meine Wasserkur* [My Water Cure] (Kempten: Kögel-Verlag, 1914).

CHAPTER 12. TREATMENT SEQUENCE

1. H. Mozer, *Brennpunkte der Krankheiten* [Flashpoint of Illnesses] (Heidelberg: Karl F. Haug Verlag, 1980).
2. Frederick Leboyer, *Birth without Violence* (Rochester, VT: Inner Traditions International, 1995).

CHAPTER 14. REACTIONS

1. H. H. Reckeweg, *Homotoxinlehre* [Teaching of Homotoxins] (Baden-Baden: Aurelia-Verlag, 1956).

CHAPTER 18. TREATMENT COMBINATIONS

1. E. Rauch, *Die Darmreinigung nach F. X. Mayr* [Intestinal Cleansing According to F. X. Mayr] (Heidelberg: Karl F. Haug Verlag, 1994).
2. E. Rauch, *Blut- und Säfte-Reinigung* [Blood and Fluid Cleansing] (Heidelberg: Karl F. Haug Verlag, 1980).
3. Kneipp, *Meine Wasserkur.*
4. A. Rosendorff, *Neue Erkenntnisse aus der Naturheilbehandlung* [New Insights from Homeopathy] (Bietigheim: Turm-Verlag, 1994).
5. L. Walb, *Die Haysche Trenn-Kost* [The "Haysch" Diet] (Heidelberg: Karl F. Haug Verlag, 1996).
6. A. Schaarschuh-Haase, *Amungs- und Lösungstherapie bei Schlafstörungen* [Breathing and Relaxation Therapies for Sleep Problems] (Bietigheim: Turm-verlag, 1993).

CHAPTER 19. FEET AND HANDS

1. M. Mességué, *Von Menschen und Pflanzen* [Of People and Plants] (Munich: Molden, 1972).

CHAPTER 23. CASE HISTORIES

1. E. Rauch, *Blut- und Säfte-Reinigung.*
2. F. Riemkasten, *Die Alexander Methode* [The Alexander Method: Meaning, Consequences and Ways to End Posture Problems] (Heidelberg: Karl F. Haug Verlag, 1999).

CHAPTER 25. INDICATIONS FOR REFLEX ZONE THERAPY

1. Rauch, *Die Darmreinigung nach F.X. Mayr and Blut- und Säfte-Reinigung.*
2. Rosendorff, *Neue Erkenntnisse aus der Naturheilbehandlung.*

Bibliography

Alexander, Gerda. *Eutonie.* Munich: Koesel, 1992.

Bressler, Harry Bond. *Zone Therapy.* Pomeroy, WA: Health Research Books, 1971.

Dicke, Elizabeth. *Meine Bindegewebsmassage* [My Connective Tissue Massage]. Stuttgart: Hippokrates Verlag, 1962.

Feldenkrais, M. *Bewusstheit durch Bewegung* [Consciousness through Movement]. Frankfurt: Suhrkamp, 1978.

Fitzgerald, William H., and Edwin F. Bowers. *Zone Therapy: Relieving Pain at Home.* Pomeroy, WA.: Health Research Books, 1994.

Helmrich, H. *Kompendium der Bindegewebsmassage* [Compendium of Connective Tissue Massage]. Heidelberg: Karl F. Haug Verlag, 1994.

Ingham, Eunice D., and Dwight Byers. *The Original Works of Eunice Ingham: Stories the Feet Can Tell thru Reflexology* and *Stories the Feet Have Told thru Reflexology.* St. Petersburg, La.: Ingham Publishing, 1984.

Kneipp, Sebastian. *Meine Wasserkur* [My Water Cure]. Kempten: Kösel-Verlag, 1914.

Leboyer, Frederic. *Birth without Violence.* Rochester, VT.: Inner Traditions International, 1995.

Mességué, M. *Von Menschen und Pflanzen* [Of People and Plants]. Munich: Molden, 1972.

Mozer, H. *Brennpunkte der Krankheiten* [Flashpoints of Illnesses]. Heidelberg: Karl F. Haug Verlag, 1980.

Palm, H. *Das gesunde Haus—unser naechster Umweltschutz.* [The Healthy House—Our Next Environmental Cause]. Konstanz: Ordo Verlag, 1992.

Pschyrembel, W. *Klinisches Wörterbuch* [Clinical Dictionary]. Berlin: Verlag Walter de Gruyter, 1998.

Rauch, E. *Die Darmreinigung nach F. X. Mayr* [Intestinal Cleansing According to F.X. Mayr]. Heidelberg: Karl F. Haug Verlag, 1994.

Rauch, E. *Blut- und Säfte-Reinigung* [Blood and Fluid Cleansing]. Heidelberg: Karl F. Haug Verlag, 1980.

Reckeweg, H. H. *Homotoxinlehre* [Teaching of Homotoxins]. Baden-Baden: Aurelia-Verlag, 1956.

Riemkasten, F. *Die Alexander Methode. Bedeutung, Folgen und Abstellung der Haltungsschaeden.* [The Alexander Method: Meaning, Consequences and Ways to End Posture Problems]. Heidelberg: Karl F. Haug Verlag, 1994.

Rosendorff, A. *Neue Erkenntnisse aus der Naturheilbehandlung* [New Insights from Homeopathy]. Bietigheim: Turm-Verlag, 1994.

Schaarschuch-Haase, A. *Atmungs und Lösungstherapie bei Schlafstörungen* [Breathing and Relaxation Therapies for Sleep Problems]. Bietigheim: Turm-Verlag, 1993.

Walb, L. *Die Haysche Trenn-Kost* [The "Haysch" Diet]. Heidelberg: Karl F. Haug Verlag, 1996.

Voll, R. *Topographic Positions of the Measurement Points in Electro-acupuncture.* Uelzen, Germany: Medizinisch Literarische Verlagsgesellschaft, 1978.

About the Author

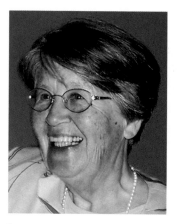

Hanne Marquardt, a registered nurse, naturopath, and student of the reflexology pioneer Eunice Ingham, is the most well-known and experienced reflexologist in Europe today.

Born in 1933, Marquardt began her nurse's training in 1951. In 1955, she became a licensed masseuse, and from 1956 to 1957, she taught at the school of massage in Boppard, Germany. In 1958, she completed her training as a respiratory therapist, passing her homeopathy exam in 1961. Through 1967 she continued to practice reflex zone therapy, primarily at her own clinic, and in 1970, she began training medical therapeutic specialists at the center in Königsfeld-Burgberg, Germany.

The founder of fifteen reflexology schools in Germany and abroad, she lectures on foot reflexology throughout the world.

Index

Page numbers in *italics* refer to illustrations.

BOOKS OF RELATED INTEREST

The Reflexology Manual
An Easy-to-Use Illustrated Guide to the Healing Zones
of the Hands and Feet
by Pauline Wills

The Reflexology Atlas
by Bernard C. Kolster, M.D., and Astrid Waskowiak, M.D.

Facial Reflexology
A Self-Care Manual
by Marie-France Muller, M.D., N.D., Ph.D.

Sexual Reflexology
Activating the Taoist Points of Love
by Mantak Chia and William U. Wei

Gemstone Reflexology
by Nora Kircher

Total Reflexology
The Reflex Points for Physical, Emotional,
and Psychological Healing
by Martine Faure-Alderson, D.O.

The Encyclopedia of Healing Points
The Home Guide to Acupoint Treatment
by Roger Dalet, M.D.

Trigger Point Therapy for Myofascial Pain
The Practice of Informed Touch
by Donna Finando, L.Ac., L.M.T., and Steven Finando, Ph.D., L.Ac.

Inner Traditions • Bear & Company
P.O. Box 388
Rochester, VT 05767
1-800-246-8648
www.InnerTraditions.com

Or contact your local bookseller